Preparing to Breastfeed:

A Pregnant Woman's Guide

By Teresa Pitman

Preparing to Breastfeeding:
A Pregnant Woman's Guide

Teresa Pitman

Hale Publishing, L.P.

1712 N. Forest St.

Amarillo, TX 79106-7017

806-376-9900

800-378-1317

www.iBreastfeeding.com

Library of Congress Control Number: 2013937661

ISBN-13: 978-1-9398473-7-9

Dedication

For Esmaralda, Alison, and Heather: My sons clearly have excellent taste.

Table of Contents

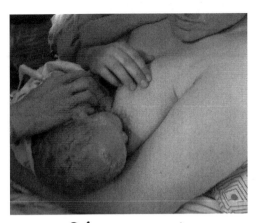

Chapter 1.
The Truth
about Breastfeeding

Most women decide how they are going to feed their babies long before they become pregnant. Sometimes it's seeing your own siblings' breastfeed – or hearing your mother talk about breastfeeding you – that nudges you in that direction. Sometimes it's seeing your friends with babies at their breasts that makes you think, hey, I could do that!

Or maybe you're bucking the trend among your family and friends by even considering breastfeeding, because most of them used formula and bottles for their babies. You might even have had some discouraging comments from them already, if you've shared your plans.

Even if you have some concerns, you're not ready to give up on your plans. You've probably heard that breastfeeding has benefits for your baby: It makes them healthier and smarter. Maybe that's even why you decided to breastfeed.

Maybe you've also heard – from your friends and family – that breastfeeding is difficult, painful, and many women don't make enough milk anyway. No worries if you have to wean, because breast is best - but formula is just as good.

Here's the truth: Breastfeeding doesn't have "benefits." It's just the biologically normal way to feed a baby. Human milk is the milk that meets the needs of human babies, providing the appropriate nutrition and, just as important, immune support so that the baby can stay healthy and develop normally. Further, lactating is what breasts are designed to do. The hormones produced when breastfeeding are normal for women in their child-bearing years, so breastfeeding mothers are protected against many illnesses and health problems.

If breastfeeding is biologically normal for babies, it's not surprising that any other way of feeding the baby has some risks. And, in fact, that's what all the research tells us: Babies who are not breastfed are at higher risk of a long list of illnesses. These babies are more likely to get:

- Respiratory illnesses, such as colds, flu, bronchitis, RSV, and pneumonia
- Infections in the stomach and intestines causing vomiting, diarrhea, and sometimes dehydration
- Necrotizing enterocolitis (an infection of the gut often fatal to premature infants)
- Ear infections
- GERD (reflux)
- Hernias
- Urinary tract infections
- Meningitis
- Other contagious diseases they may be exposed to
- Type 1 diabetes
- Type 2 diabetes
- Some childhood cancers
- High blood pressure and heart disease (as adults)
- Celiac disease
- Crohn's disease or ulcerative colitis
- Asthma
- Eczema
- Rheumatoid arthritis
- Multiple sclerosis
- Breast cancer (for girls, when they are adults)

They are more than twice as likely to die of SIDS.

They are more likely to be overweight or obese as children and as adults.

They are more likely to have malocclusions (teeth that need braces or other orthodontic work) and to need speech therapy to help them speak clearly.

They are more likely to have anxiety, depression, and other mental health problems as children and teens.

If their mothers are depressed, babies who are not breastfed are more likely to have developmental changes in their brains and to experience depression later. When babies of depressed mothers are breastfed, their brains develop normally.

They are likely to have lower IQs and lower achievement scores in school than those who are breastfed.

They are more likely to die in their first year from all causes.

The mother who does not breastfeed is more likely to:

- Have a post-partum hemorrhage.

- Develop Type 2 diabetes.

- Be overweight or obese later in life.

- Become anemic.

- Develop osteoporosis.

- Develop endometriosis.

- Develop uterine cancer.

- Develop ovarian cancer.

- Develop breast cancer.

Wow. That's quite a long list of risks that babies (and their mothers) are exposed to when they are not breastfed. That doesn't mean that some breastfed babies don't get sick – of course they do! And some babies fed formula will be lucky enough to stay healthy and avoid all these risks. But the research – and there is a substantial body of research on these issues now – is clear that not breastfeeding increases your baby's chances of getting many illnesses and can affect his psychological and intellectual development.

But Is the Research Reliable?

You might have heard that these studies are not really reliable. Some writers have pointed out that most of the mothers in North America who breastfeed have more education and higher socio-economic status than the mothers who don't breastfeed (Ingall, 2006). (Not always true, but statistically that's the case.) So perhaps the breastfed babies are healthier just because babies of better-educated, wealthier parents are pretty much always healthier – thanks to the families' better nutrition and access to medical care. Maybe it's not the breastfeeding at all.

The "standard" for good research is the randomized, double-blind study. Obviously, you can't just do randomized studies and assign half the mothers to breastfeed and half to not breastfeed. Mothers won't stand for it! And you can't make the study "blind" either – mothers know if they are breastfeeding or not! But there have been studies that tried to approach these questions with some variation of randomization.

One study looked at premature babies who were being fed through a tube that went directly into their stomach (Lucas, Morley, Cole, Lister, & Leeson-Payne, 1992). These babies were randomly assigned to be given either human milk or formula in those tube-feedings. Eight years later, the babies who had received human milk scored significantly higher on IQ tests than those who had received formula.

Another study considered the differences between babies born in "Baby-Friendly" hospitals and those born in hospitals that were not "Baby-Friendly" (Kramer et al., 2008). (I'll discuss the "Baby-Friendly Hospital Initiative" in more detail later in the book, but the short version is that it is a program where hospitals follow certain steps to support breastfeeding.) The communities where the hospitals were located were similar, and had similar breastfeeding rates before the hospital went Baby-Friendly. After the Baby-Friendly steps were initiated, the rates of breastfeeding among the babies born in the Baby-Friendly hospitals were much higher. The other factors (wealth, education, etc.) were still similar among the communities, so this made for a good comparison. And, in fact, the researchers found that on average the babies born in the Baby-Friendly hospitals had lower rates of many diseases, as well as higher scores on tests of intelligence and development.

So what's so important about breastfeeding? Most of the research that was done just looked at the numbers – how many formula-fed babies got sick compared to how many breastfed babies got sick – but newer research is starting to look at *how* breastmilk provides protection against diseases.

For example, one recent study discovered that when babies digested formula (but not human milk), a toxin was produced that actually destroyed some of the cells in the baby's intestines (Penn et al., 2012). This may be a major reason why premature babies fed formula are so much more likely to develop necrotizing enterocolitis. In full-term and healthy babies, their bodies seem to be better able to eliminate these toxins – but really, it's better not to have them in your system at all.

Researchers have found that human milk is loaded with antibodies (from the mother's system) and other factors that boost the baby's immune system. When the baby nurses, the milk coats his mouth, throat, and stomach – creating a barrier of live, active antibodies that stop the germs from getting into the baby's body. The immune factors pass into the bloodstream and encourage the baby to produce his own antibodies. (And if the baby spits up a bit, or gets milk up his nose, that's a good thing – the antibodies go to work in yet another part of the body!)

Because the mother and baby are usually sharing the same environment, these antibodies are perfectly individualized for the baby's needs. If they are out at the park together, and another child sneezes in their direction, the mom's body will quickly start making antibodies to fight whatever virus was in that sneeze – and will share those antibodies with the baby through her milk. The antibodies are constantly changing in response to the environment.

As well, other immune factors in the milk stimulate the baby's system to produce his own antibodies and gear up to fight the infection.

Researchers who were doing studies to see how long human milk could be left at room temperature tried injecting bacteria into samples of milk (Marks, Clementi, & Hakansson, 2012). They wanted to see how quickly the milk would be contaminated by the bacteria and spoiled. What they found was that the antibodies in the milk actually killed the bacteria. Now, that doesn't mean you can leave your milk out for too long – eventually the live antibodies will begin to die off and the bacteria will start to reproduce. But the studies found that human milk can quite safely be left at room temperature for six to eight hours, and in a fridge for five days. Don't try that with formula!

Studies also found that the process of digesting formula puts added stress on the baby's body (Jorgenson, Ott, Juul, Skakkebaek, & Michaelsen, 2003). Because there are more toxins and waste products that need to be removed when a baby is consuming formula, his liver and kidneys are working harder than the breastfed baby's organs are. That may mean fewer reserves to fight off infections and diseases.

Remember that formula is based on cow's milk, and cow's milk is intended for baby calves – who need to grow very quickly and who aren't especially intelligent. Human milk is designed to meet the slower growth needs of human babies and promote brain development.

The Joys of Breastfeeding

Of course, on a day-to-day basis, these aren't the things breastfeeding mothers think about. When you're nursing your baby for the 10th time that day, you're not congratulating yourself for reducing your risk of osteoporosis or helping your baby develop better jaw structure. No, mostly you're just thinking, "When will I get some sleep??"

But there are a lot of ways that breastfeeding makes mothering easier, too. Not so much in the beginning, when you and your baby are both learning. But learning any new skill is like that. If you drive a car, you may remember what it was like when you started out. You had to think through every step – key in ignition, which way do you turn it? Which pedal is the gas again? Your driving was often jerky and bumpy, and sometimes you went too fast and sometimes too slow. You'd feel exhausted after just driving to the mall, because it took so much concentration. After a few weeks, though, driving became second nature. You could carry on a conversation, listen to the radio, make a mental list of what you needed to buy, and still drive safely through the streets. Your feet automatically went to the right pedals when you needed to stop or speed up, without any conscious thought.

Learning to breastfeed is much the same. Sometimes there are challenges at the beginning and it seems like a lot to remember. But soon it's so easy you barely think about it.

And the hormones that go along with milk production help you in other ways. A 2011 study examined MRIs of mothers' brains while they listened to their babies crying (Kim et al., 2011). The researchers found that when breastfeeding mothers hear their babies' cry, the parts of their brains that are linked to nurturing and empathetic and responsive behavior are more likely to light up. When mothers who are not breastfeeding hear those cries, they don't have as much activity in these parts of their brains. The researchers also found that the mothers with more of that response in their brain showed more sensitive and caring behavior with their babies.

Now, that doesn't mean a mother who uses formula can't be a good mother. An earlier study which found similar results followed the mothers over time and found that the non-breastfeeding mothers did develop a more nurturing brain response after a few months of caring for their babies (Swain, Lorberbaum, Kose, & Strathearn, 2007). But those breastfeeding hormones can sure help you during those early challenging weeks.

Breastfeeding – when it is going well – also helps reduce the risk of post-partum depression or negative mood. You might have heard the opposite – maybe you've had a friend who was encouraged to stop breastfeeding because she was depressed. And it's true that if a mother is having serious problems with breastfeeding (sore nipples or a baby who is having difficulty latching) that can make her feel stressed and anxious, and add to her depression. All the more reason to start preparing early and to make sure you have some good help lined up for when your baby is born!

Once you get breastfeeding going well, you start to notice all the other good reasons to breastfeed:

- Breastfeeding is better for the environment – no cans or plastic bags to throw away, no pollution from manufacturing companies, no gas used to transport to the stores or to your home, no waste products to pollute the water. It's the epitome of "eat local!"

- Breastfeeding is inexpensive. Yes, there are people who will try to sell you special nursing pillows, bras, pumps, and other equipment, but the reality is that you generally don't need any of that. You've got breasts, you've got a baby – you're all set. You might find you need to eat a little bit more – about the equivalent of an extra peanut butter sandwich each day – but that will cost you far less than the many cans of infant formula a formula-fed baby will go through, and also save you the cost of gas to drive to the store and buy the formula, bottles, etc.

- The hormones of breastfeeding calm and comfort you. Research shows that breastfeeding mothers are less likely to be depressed or to feel stressed and anxious. And if you are – put your baby to the breast and feel those hormones relax you!

- Breastfed babies have bowel movements that don't smell as bad. (One father of a breastfed baby visited a friend whose baby was formula fed and was shocked to realize how much worse his poopy diapers smelled.) That may be a small thing, but you will be changing many, many diapers!

- Breastfed babies themselves smell better – sweeter and fresher.

- Breastfeeding soothes babies. If your baby is hungry, thirsty, lonely, scared, in pain – breastfeeding will comfort him.

- In an emergency situation – when a winter storm knocks out the power for several days or hurricane damage means clean water is unavailable for a period of time – breastfeeding remains safe. Formula is only safe if you have access to clean water (for preparation of powdered formula and for cleaning bottles and nipples) and of course can't provide any protection against the diseases that may be a problem during these emergency situations. Human milk is not only safe (in fact, as mentioned earlier, it actively kills bacteria), but it will help protect the baby against any contagious diseases that might be around.

Here's what some breastfeeding mothers have said about their experiences:

Sue Ann Kendall – "I loved that breastfeeding instantly calmed an upset baby. If they were hurt or sad, it helped. Plus I could help immediately when they were hungry. They did not sit there and cry, waiting for me to prepare formula."

Anna Baker – "I love how breastfeeding connects me to my body and my instincts, and makes me slow down. I had a lot of anxiety and insomnia during my son's first year, and I remember so clearly the calming rush of hormones that come with breastfeeding and skin-to-skin cuddles. Sometimes if I couldn't sleep, I offered the breast just to help settle myself down! And now, nursing a three-year-old, I'm still grateful for the connection nursing brings – not only with my boy, but with my body and heart."

Saara Murnick – "I loved knowing that I was all my little ones needed. It made me trust my body when I saw them thriving. I didn't look at clocks, or how much I could pump (never much) – I just had to see that they were growing and happy, and I was content. For the tough parts, the support of other La Leche League moms and my own mom – their knowledge and availability – was what got me through. As for what I wish I'd known? I guess the only thing that shocked me was when my second son came along and it wasn't a cake walk. I figured that I'd already breastfed one child into toddlerhood, and I knew how to do it... but what I didn't take into account is that every child is different, and I'd forgotten how to breastfeed a newborn. It was a learning experience for both of us until we figured out what would work for us. Even with past experience, every child is different and every nursing relationship is different."

Linda Whitehill Anderegg – "I think what I loved most was when my son would look into my eyes and break into a big grin, and milk would come dribbling out the corners of his mouth, knowing that me and my body were making him so happy. I remember the pride I felt watching my scrawny little baby fill out and almost double his weight at about eight weeks. It was a wonderful time in my life after those first two rough weeks were over. I loved every minute of nursing him."

Becky Kaye – "Being cheap and lazy, I loved the fact that it was free and always the right temperature, and no bottles to wash and sterilize! My babies were completely portable because the food was always at the ready! I loved being needed and the feeling of satisfaction that came with not only creating a wonderful new human being, but being able to provide sustenance from my body as well. I thought I would feel overwhelmed and tied down by this, but I didn't, knowing it wouldn't last forever. Especially with my youngest, I enjoyed the middle of the night feedings when it was quiet – so peaceful and tranquil – I could feel, see, and hear the nourishment that I gave him. So powerful!"

But Isn't It Hard?

So – it's good for your baby. Good for you. And moms love it. After reading all that, I'm hoping you're motivated to give breastfeeding a try. But maybe now you're feeling a little nervous. Your sister wanted to breastfeed her baby, but ended up in tears because of the pain and turned to formula. Your friend had hoped to breastfeed, but soon had to supplement, and within weeks found her baby preferred the bottle to her breast and refused to nurse any more. Is this really going to work for you?

Let's be honest. Some women are not able to produce a full milk supply for their babies. (We'll talk more about why this might happen, what alternatives you have, and some indications to keep in mind to know if this might be the case for you in later chapters.) Some babies have difficulty breastfeeding for a variety of reasons, including anatomical problems, such as cleft palates. In many of these cases, you may be able to pump or express your milk and give it to your baby some other way. These situations can be very frustrating and disappointing, and it only makes it worse when people say, "Oh, all mothers can breastfeed." Not true.

But – and this is a big BUT – the vast majority of the cases where women struggle with breastfeeding happen because the mothers get off to a rough start and don't get the help they need.

For proof of that, we only need to look at the situation in other countries. Statistics can be very revealing:

- In Canada, 85% of mothers start out breastfeeding their babies, but 27% of those mothers stop within the first four weeks. Only 23% exclusively breastfeed for at least six months (the current recommendation of the Canadian Pediatric Society and the World Health Organization; Health Canada, 2012).

- In the U.S., about 77% of mothers start out breastfeeding, only 36% are still breastfeeding at three months, and only 16% breastfeed exclusively for six months (Centers for Disease Control and Prevention, 2012). The American Academy of Pediatrics also recommends exclusive breastfeeding for six months. These recommendations don't mean that breastfeeding should stop at six months! Not at all! That's just the point where solid foods can be added to the babies' diet, with recommendations for continued breastfeeding for two years and beyond.

- In Norway, 97% of women start out breastfeeding, and about 80% are still exclusively breastfeeding at six months (Kellymom.com, 2012).

- In Madagascar, almost 100% of women start out breastfeeding, and 54% are still exclusively breastfeeding at six months (Childinfo, 2013). The rest are still breastfeeding, but have added solid foods.

Are women and babies in Canada and the U.S. that different from mothers and babies in Norway and Madagascar? I think what these wide variations show are not biological differences, but differences in support and attitudes.

In Norway, for example, most women give birth with midwives, and the midwives consider being able to help with breastfeeding an essential part of their skill-set. Mothers are cared for by midwives during their pregnancies, during the birth, and for several weeks afterwards. Norway also provides significant paid maternity leave for new mothers.

Norway has also banned advertising of infant formulas to parents.

Breastfeeding is even encouraged and promoted for premature or ill babies. Midwife Rachel Myr, who works in Norway, describes the process in her hospital when a baby needing extra care is born:

> The NICU (Neonatal Intensive Care Unit) have what they call 'kangaroo admission.' For premature babies, babies of diabetic mothers, or any baby who needs close monitoring but no technical life support systems, the baby is administratively a patient of the NICU while s/he stays with mother, on her body, and a NICU nurse comes to the birthing room to observe the baby from birth, feed it donor milk if mother is diabetic (to avoid plummeting blood glucose which might necessitate admission to the physical NICU), and do whatever other monitoring is necessitated by the baby's condition. The NICU nurse continues to care

for the baby after mother and baby come to postpartum together. Best of both worlds - mothers and babies stay together, staff on postpartum can support mother, and the NICU nurse makes sure baby is OK by being present to a degree our own staffing simply doesn't allow. Parents LOVE it. Naturally, the babies are happy and more stable, and breastfeeding is easier. We can care for the mother more easily because she is totally present as long as the baby is with her. It is such a change – instead of this distressed facial expression on the mother because she is so far away from her baby, or just never finding her in her room to see what she needs from us, we come in and find everyone looking deliriously happy.

In Madagascar, as in Norway, there is strong support from society for breastfeeding. Women feel comfortable breastfeeding in public and have experienced friends and family to turn to if they have questions or need help. Because breastfeeding is treated as normal, it works most of the time.

In the U.S. and Canada (and many other countries), many women who want to breastfeed don't get off to a good start. They may get unhelpful advice in the hospital or from family and friends who don't have much experience. Once they get home, it can get worse: Knowledgeable help can be hard to find (many doctors know very little about breastfeeding), friends and relatives can be more discouraging than helpful, and breastfeeding in public draws stares and rude comments.

And just when you're at your lowest point, a free case of formula arrives on your doorstep, or formula coupons come in the mail, or you see a commercial on TV asking you, "What makes a happy mom? A happy feeding!" The message: Just give your baby our formula and all will be well. It's not surprising that many mothers end up weaning sooner than they wanted to.

Another difference: In Canada, epidural rates range from 30% to 69% depending on the province, and C-section rates are between 23% and 29% (Canadian Institute for Health Information, 2013). In the U.S., epidural rates average 61% and C-sections are at 31% (VBAC.com, 2013). In Norway, fewer than 25% of the mothers have epidurals in labor and about 14% have C-sections (Tveit, Halvorsen, & Rosland, 2009). Birth *does* affect breastfeeding.

Remember that even if your own mother didn't breastfeed – or didn't breastfeed for long – you are still the product of a long line of breastfeeding mothers. If you could travel back in time a few hundred years, you'd find that breastfeeding was pretty close to 100 percent, although a few of the wealthiest families used wet nurses, so the mothers' fertility would return more quickly. Those are your ancestors. Breastfeeding has always been so important to the human race that it tends to work even in very tough situations.

With good information and some support, you can feel confident that – like those mothers in Norway and Madagascar – you will be able to get breastfeeding off to a good start and keep going as long as you want (even if you face some challenges along the way).

What You Can Do Now

1. Write down the risks of not breastfeeding that are most significant to you. Ask your partner to do the same. Knowing why breastfeeding is important to you can help you keep going if you have some challenging times.

2. Are there some situations you think might be potential barriers for you? Breastfeeding in public? Negative reactions from family or friends? Needing to return to work? Make a list of these concerns and see if you can think of ways to resolve them or reduce the impact of the problem. You may want to talk to other mothers who have dealt with these concerns to find out what they did.

3. Who do you think will be your cheerleaders for breastfeeding? Who will support and encourage you when you need it? Make a list of those people as well, and keep it handy!

4. Consider attending a La Leche League meeting in your community. (To find one, you can check www.lllc.ca (Canada) or (www.llli.org.) It's a great way to learn about breastfeeding, meet other mothers (every meeting is different, but you can usually expect pregnant women, mothers with new babies, and mothers with older babies or toddlers to be there), and establish contacts with people who can help you if you do have questions or concerns once your baby is born.

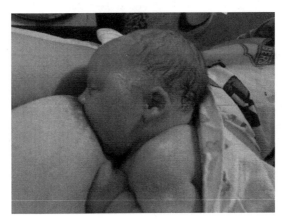

Chapter 2.
How Breastfeeding Works

It can seem like a mysterious – maybe even magical – process. You have a baby and your breasts start making milk to feed them, something they've never done before. How does that happen? We're learning more and more about what goes on inside our bodies as researchers use new technology to better understand the physiology and biology of breastfeeding. While it's certainly not essential to know all the technical terms (and I'm not going to use many here!), a basic understanding of how the process works can help you solve breastfeeding problems and figure out how to handle challenging situations.

Even if you weren't planning to breastfeed, your breasts will be. In fact, they've been working up to the day when they start providing nutrition for your baby for a very long time – since puberty.

The Beginnings of Breasts

When your breasts begin to develop at around age ten, part of what happens is that additional fat tissue is laid down. That's what gives your breasts their appealing shape and size. But while that's the visible change, that's not all that is going on. A network of ducts is also growing beneath the surface, connecting milk-producing glands near your chest wall and underarms with your nipple. A similar network of blood vessels develops, too, to provide the nutrients needed when it's time to make milk.

Then, as puberty ends, your breasts go into waiting mode. They wait. And wait. And wait for the day when those pregnancy hormones start circulating throughout your system. At last all those ducts and special cells are ready to spring into action.

The Pregnant Breast

Once you are pregnant, your breasts quickly get into high gear. (If you've been on birth control pills that mimic pregnancy in order to prevent conception, your breasts may have responded to those hormones and already started this phase of development.) That basic network of ducts laid down many years ago isn't going to be enough to really sustain a baby – that was just the foundation. With a pregnancy underway, new ducts will grow and new connections will be built. The milk-producing glands multiply and get ready to go into production. Your nipples and the skin around them (called the areolas) will often darken in color (depending on how dark they were pre-pregnancy), ready to attract the eye of your new baby. You will grow new veins – in fact, you can often see them as blue lines under the skin of your breasts – ready to support milk production.

All this growth and change can make your breasts rather tender and sensitive during the first few months of pregnancy. Sometimes it even hurts to have the water from the shower run on your breasts! You may find you need bras with a larger cup size as well. That's normal – in fact, it's an excellent sign that your breasts are getting ready to feed your baby.

By seven months or so, your breasts aren't just getting ready, they are often actively producing milk, although in small amounts. You may see the thick, yellowish droplets after you have a shower or notice that you are leaking a little milk during sex (or the prelude to sex). If you squeeze your breast behind your nipple, you might get more drops or even a little spray of milk. Some women don't really notice any milk at this stage, and that's okay too. This early milk is called colostrum. This milk will be your baby's first food, and it's powerful stuff – full of antibodies and nutrients ideal for your newborn.

Because you are still pregnant, you only make small quantities of this first milk. The pregnancy hormones produced by the placenta prevent milk production from increasing to the levels your baby will need later.

Breasts, Meet Baby

Once your baby is born, though, and the placenta delivered, the pregnancy hormones disappear. Now milk production really gets underway. It takes typically two or three days (depending in part on how often your baby nurses) for your milk volume to increase after the baby is born.

During the first few days of your baby's life, you'll still be making that beautiful and very valuable colostrum. It's a concentrated and highly nutritious milk, loaded with antibodies and anti-infective properties, that is designed to coat your baby's stomach and intestinal tract, protecting him from any germs that might want to get into his system. It's also a laxative, so it helps to clean out the meconium (the black stool that is in the baby's intestines before birth), reducing the risk of jaundice. And it has plenty of protein and easily digested sugars to keep your baby's blood sugar stable. You don't want your baby to miss out on this!

Yes, you only produce small amounts of colostrum, but that's not a big deal. At this stage, your baby's tummy is the size of a chickpea. That's tiny! It doesn't take much to fill him up, but because he's also trying to grow quickly (and looking for comfort and soothing in this brand new world he's just been born into), he'll come back again for another feeding soon. Those frequent feedings have another purpose, as I'll explain later.

All these things we've just described will happen whether or not you have chosen to breastfeed. Your breasts will grow a wonderful system of milk ducts, start producing colostrum, and increase the milk volume after a few days, even if you never put your baby to the breast and never intend to.

But at this point, milk production starts to be affected by what you and your baby do.

Building Milk Production

In the first few days, your breasts are learning about what's needed. You might have had one petite baby who doesn't need a large volume of milk. Or you might have had triplets! Most women start out with an oversupply of milk – at least enough to feed twins – and over the first days and weeks, the amount produced is adjusted by how often the baby nurses and how much milk he takes at each feeding.

During these early feedings, receptors that are sensitive to the hormones that boost milk production are formed in the milk-producing areas of the breast. If there are relatively infrequent feedings taking small amounts of milk each time, fewer receptors grow. This might be the situation if you had just one baby who was destined to be on the small side. If there are frequent feedings taking a substantial amount of milk each time, more receptors are laid down. This would be the case if you had hungry triplets!

These receptors will roughly determine how much milk your breasts will produce down the road. Your milk supply can be adjusted upwards and (more easily) downwards later, but if there are fewer receptors, it can sometimes be harder to increase your milk production later on. That's why those early weeks and days are so important: You want to be sure your breasts get the right messages!

But How Is Milk Actually Made?

Without getting too technical about the process, milk is made from your blood. As the blood passes by the milk-making cells in your breasts, the nutrients, antibodies, immune factors, and other ingredients needed for your baby are extracted and deposited in precise proportions into the ducts. The fat that is moved from your bloodstream into the milk is in round globules that float freely in the milk, but tend to stick to the sides of the ducts.

The milk usually waits in the "back" part of your breasts (closer to your ribcage) until the muscles around the ducts contract and push the milk towards the nipple. We call this the milk "letting down." (The sensation of the baby nursing can cause those contractions and the milk "letdown" that results – or it can happen when you just think about your baby, or smell his clothes, or hear him cry...) In the early weeks, this control system doesn't always work well, and mothers may find they leak milk throughout the day, or just before feedings. Usually, the leaking stops after six weeks or so (although some women experience leaking for a longer period of time).

But there is another important thing that goes on while the milk is in the "waiting room." The more milk that is sitting around, the more pressure there is on the walls of the duct. This pressure signals the milk-making cells to slow down and cut back on the amount of milk being produced. It's the "feedback loop" that adjusts milk supply.

When the milk is removed quickly, there is little pressure on the duct walls, and the milk-making process is speeded up.

What this means to you: The emptier your breast is, the more milk you make and the more quickly you make it. The fuller your breast is, the less milk you make and the more slowly you make it. Over time, this will reduce milk production.

This is one reason that stretching out the time between feedings, or trying to wait until your breasts "fill up" with milk before feeding, or scheduling feedings all tend to lead to breastfeeding problems. These approaches all decrease milk production. Frequent feedings, on the other hand, keep the breasts always partially empty, encouraging the glands to keep production revved up.

Another factor in making sure you have plenty of milk: When you breastfeed at night, your body produces higher levels of the hormone that stimulates milk production. So those night feedings are important not just for satisfying your baby's hunger tonight, but for making sure you'll have plenty of milk to give her tomorrow and the next day.

And yet another factor: Skin-to-skin contact with your baby, even if the baby isn't breastfeeding, also seems to promote milk production. Being skin-to-skin with you has many benefits for your baby, including reducing stress, maintaining temperature, stabilizing heart rate and breathing, and raising blood sugar levels if they are low. Another win-win!

Murphy's Law: What Can Go Wrong? And How Can We Prevent It?

Breastfeeding is a complex system on the inside, yet it seems very simple in action. It works remarkably well in a wide variety of situations with two important caveats: Mother and baby are kept together (ideally with maximum skin-to-skin contact) and baby is able to nurse effectively as often as needed.

When these basics get messed up, you may have problems.

Here's one example: A British researcher, Helen Ball, divided a group of breastfeeding mothers who had just given birth into three groups (Ball, Ward-Platt, Heslop, Leech, & Brown, 2006). They were all in the same hospital. The first group had their babies in a bassinet beside the bed. The second group had their babies in bed with them. And the third group used a "co-sleeper attachment" attached to the side of the bed for the baby to sleep in (the baby was level with the bed and near the mother, but not actually in the bed). Video cameras were installed to record what happened day and night.

The researchers found that the babies who were in the bed with their mothers breastfed *twice* as often as those who were in bassinets beside the beds – even though all three groups said they were feeding on demand. The babies in the co-sleeper attachments fed slightly less often than those who were in the bed next to their mothers, but more often than those in the bassinets.

Interesting, sure, but the really important point came when the researchers followed up with the mothers four months later: Twice as many of the babies who had shared their mothers' beds in the early days were still breastfeeding compared to those who had been in the bassinet. The babies in the co-sleepers were slightly less likely to be still breastfeeding than those who had bed-shared. And the main reason for weaning? Not enough milk.

So keeping mothers and babies together means – REALLY together. Apparently (and other researchers have found similar results), either babies are less likely to signal that they need to nurse when they aren't in contact with their mothers, or mothers are less likely to pick up on baby's signals when they are even a few feet apart. Those less-frequent feedings mean milk production really doesn't get going as well as it should.

Sometimes mothers and babies are more drastically separated. A mother who has a fever (possibly as the result of having an epidural – it's a fairly common side-effect) may have her baby taken to the nursery while she is tested to be sure she's not contagious. Or the baby may be ill or premature or at risk for other reasons and need to be in a special care nursery, or may be unable to breastfeed effectively.

In any of those situations, frequent hand-expression of your milk, followed by pumping once the volume of milk increases, can imitate what your baby would be doing if he could. Frequency is important – remember that your goal is to prevent the breasts from feeling full and signaling the milk ducts to slow down. It's much more effective to pump 12 times a day for ten minutes at a time than six times a day for 20 minutes at a time.

And What About the Latch?

Ah, the latch. Most pregnant women who are planning to breastfeed have heard about the importance of getting the baby well latched on. I will go into more detail about this in later chapters, but here's why it matters: In order to effectively get milk from the breast, the baby needs to have not just the nipple in his mouth, but part of the breast as well.

There are a couple of reasons for this. One is that the ducts that expand and fill with milk are located beyond the nipple, in the breast tissue under the darker circle that is the areola, and sometimes even further back in the breast (women vary a lot in how large their areolas are). The nursing baby compresses those ducts, sending milk into his mouth. The ducts also contract in response to the mother's letdown reflex, which is triggered by the baby's suckling. But that's not the whole story. The baby also gets milk by suction, and in order for that to work he has to have a good "seal" with his mouth around the breast. When all of that is working, the baby will get the maximum amount of milk that's available.

If the latch isn't good, though, the baby can spend long periods of time at the breast, but get very little milk. Because he's not compressing the ducts effectively, he's only getting the milk that flows from the letdown – the amount that might leak out if he wasn't on the breast. This can be hugely frustrating for the mother who feels she's breastfeeding constantly, only to see that her baby's not gaining well or is even losing weight.

Often when this happens, the mother assumes that the problem must be that she's not making enough milk. Of course, in some situations this is the case, but more often the mother *is* making lots of milk – the baby just can't get it! In time, of course, the mother's milk supply will go down because her breasts are staying full even after these long and frequent feedings.

Being latched on well also means the mother will feel comfortable and not go through the pain of sore or damaged nipples. Nipples hurt when the baby isn't latched on properly, whether because his position at the breast isn't quite right or because he has some kind of anatomical difference (such as a tongue-tie) that makes it impossible for him to latch the way he needs to.

If you are experiencing any of these issues (baby nursing frequently but not gaining weight, breasts still feeling very full even after the baby has nursed, sore nipples), get in touch with a knowledgeable breastfeeding expert as soon as possible. He or she will be able to help you with the baby's latch, if that is the issue, or identify other possible problems.

Do All Breasts Make the Same Amount of Milk?

The answer to this appears to be no. Some women, as we have mentioned previously, have difficulty producing a full milk supply, even if they get great help and do everything "right." This is usually because their breasts didn't develop as expected.

Most other women will make plenty of milk for their babies if they get off to a good start and develop that capacity. But women are different in another way. Some women can store more milk in the ducts in their breasts than others. Women with more storage capacity can give the baby more milk at each feeding; women with smaller storage capacity can make just as much milk over 24 hours, but they provide less at each feeding. Ultrasound studies have been able to clearly identify these differences.

It's as though some women are feeding their babies with four-ounce bottles, and others are feeding them with two-ounce bottles. They can both give their babies the milk they need, but the mother using two-ounce bottles will need to feed her baby more frequently. That's why some breastfeeding mothers will say that they only breastfeed every three or four hours and their babies grow well and flourish, and others say that their babies need to nurse every two hours in order to grow well. They are both right: The mothers just have different milk storage capacities.

Knowing this, it should be clear why following feeding schedules seems to work okay for some women and their babies, and not at all for others. It's not because your baby is "spoiled" or more demanding – it's because your breasts are not the same as any other mother's, and your baby needs to adjust his feeding pattern to match your milk storage capacity.

Another interesting fact about milk production is that the amount of milk a mother produces in 24 hours doesn't increase much after the first couple of months, even though the baby keeps growing and may weigh significantly more by the time he's six or seven months. How does this work? We don't really know. The theory is that the baby gets better at digesting the milk and extracting the nutrients (and some breastfed babies will have fewer bowel movements as they get older), but we aren't certain if that's correct. We just know that it works: Breastfed babies do continue to grow well and gain weight, even while the amount of milk they get stays about the same.

Babies who are fed formula, on the other hand, need to be given more and more formula as they grow. This may be one reason that formula-fed babies are more likely to become obese: They become accustomed to the pattern of always getting more and more food. While breastfed babies are often heavier than their formula-fed friends in the early months, by the time they reach 12 months, the formula-fed baby tends to be heavier and fatter, while the breastfed baby has become leaner.

So – What Does This Mean if I Have Problems?

Whatever problems you run into (if you do), keep this understanding of how breastfeeding works in mind.

Here's one example of a mother who ran into an unexpected challenge:

> Esmaralda's first baby, Sebastian, was born at 32 weeks. That's eight weeks early, and this little guy (weighing just over four pounds) had lungs that weren't really developed enough to breathe. He spent his first week attached to a respirator that helped him get the oxygen he needed, and nutrients were fed directly into his bloodstream.
>
> But Esmaralda wanted to breastfeed and, fortunately, had a La Leche League Leader to help her with information and suggestions. When tiny Sebastian was whisked away to the

nursery soon after his birth, she asked for a sterile container and began hand-expressing her milk. She kept on hand expressing every two or three hours during those early days, or more often if she could. Hand expressing is better than using a breast pump in the first couple of days. Colostrum is thicker and "stickier" than later milk, so it tends to stick to the tubing of the pump, and because you only get a little at a time, you may end up with only a drop or two in the container. When you express by hand, you get more colostrum, and just as importantly, you can collect it all on a spoon or in a small container, without losing any in the process.

Esmaralda stored the milk she expressed in the hospital nursery fridge and found that by the time Sebastian was strong enough to breathe on his own and able to be fed, she had a substantial supply of colostrum to give him.

And by this point, her milk volume had increased. She switched to using the pump and continued to pump frequently, day and night. The hospital nurses told her that there was no point in pumping at night, and she might as well get more sleep. They pointed out that she was already making more milk than Sebastian needed; and every day, more milk was added to the stash in the nursery freezer.

But Esmaralda wasn't just pumping for that day. She wanted to breastfeed long-term – as all the health organizations recommend – and she knew that her later milk production depended on frequent removal of milk from her breasts now. She also knew that pumping at night would help with milk production.

Sebastian might only be taking a few ounces a day at this point, but within weeks he'd be ready for more, and she wanted to make sure he got what he needed.

Esmaralda kept on pumping at night and throughout the day. Sebastian was being fed through a tube that took the milk directly into his stomach, but Esmaralda made sure she was there for every feeding, and held him skin-to-skin as he was given her milk. Because he was hooked up to monitors for his heart rate, respiration, and temperature, it was obvious to everyone that he was calmer and more stable when held close to his mother. She kept him skin-to-skin as much as possible between feedings as well, and soon noticed that he was showing signs of wanting to latch on to the breast.

By the time he went home, four weeks after his birth, Sebastian was happily feeding at the breast. He never had even a drop of formula, and Esmaralda always had plenty of milk for him. Even though he wasn't capable of breastfeeding at first, she'd made sure to build up her milk production right from the start and kept on removing milk, so that her breasts got the message to keep up her supply.

He continued to breastfeed and by four months was a plump, round-cheeked little boy who nobody would have guessed had been born prematurely. He eventually weaned himself at around three years of age.

By keeping in mind the principles of how breastfeeding is established and how a good milk supply is maintained, Esmaralda was able to breastfeed despite her baby's challenging start.

Every new baby – and every situation – is unique, but knowing the basics of how to make the milk your baby needs will help you figure out strategies that work in your situation.

What You Can Do Now

1. Was any of the information in this chapter surprising to you? Is it different from information you've been told by others? You may want to think about how this might change (or reinforce) your plans for how you will breastfeed and how you will take care of the baby.

2. You might want to think over the stories you've heard from other women who have struggled with breastfeeding. Does understanding more about how breastfeeding works help you better understand what might have gone wrong for them? Do you have some ideas now about how you can avoid those problems?

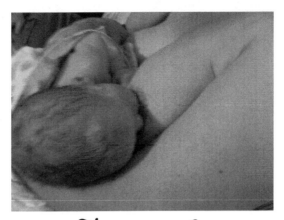

Chapter 3.
The Personal History of Your Breasts

Everyone's breasts are a little different. In fact, each of your breasts will be unique: One will be a little larger, or your nipples will be at slightly different angles, or the size and shape of the areolas will vary. That's normal, and breasts of all shapes and all sizes can produce plenty of milk and work well for breastfeeding. (The nurse who looked at my chest after my first baby was born and said, "You have the wrong kind of breasts for breastfeeding" was WRONG.)

Before you got pregnant, you probably just thought of these things in terms of how your breasts looked. Maybe it was a bit awkward to find a bra that fit well because your breasts are different sizes, or maybe someone once commented on how large your nipples are. Now with breastfeeding in mind, you're moving beyond form to function. You're looking at your breasts in a whole new way.

And the truth is that there are some aspects of breast development and the history of your breasts that can create extra challenges in breastfeeding. Some women will not be able to produce enough milk to meet all their baby's needs because of the way their breasts developed or because of health issues or past surgery. This can be very discouraging news for the mother who really wants to nurse her baby, but knowing about potential problems can help you plan and make sure you have extra help available when you need it. And, fortunately, there are good ways to supplement the baby with donated human milk (or formula, if human milk is not available), so you can continue to breastfeed while making sure your baby gets all the calories and nutrition he needs.

Even if you can't breastfeed exclusively with your own milk, you can still breastfeed.

So let's take a look at some of the ways your breasts are unique and what this might mean for breastfeeding.

Nipples

Nipple Size

There are wide variations in normal nipple size and shape. Some women have small, fairly flat nipples. Others have large, protruding nipples, and everyone else is somewhere in between. For the most part, they're all good. But sometimes there are challenges...

Small Nipples

Many women with small and/or flat nipples worry that their babies will have a hard time latching on to them. They look at the large, firm, rubber nipple on a baby bottle, realize their own nipples look and feel NOTHING like that – so how can they possibly work? Don't worry, they'll work just fine. Remember that getting milk from a baby bottle is very different from breastfeeding. The baby being fed with a bottle is getting milk primarily by sucking, with some help from gravity, and he's taking only the nipple into his mouth. The baby at the breast, on the other hand, gets milk partially through suction, but also by compressing the ducts within the breast, and from the mother's milk-ejection reflex. And you'll notice that it's called "breastfeeding," not "nipple-feeding." That's because the baby takes a good mouthful of breast, as well as the nipple, into his mouth as he nurses. The ducts he needs to compress are in the breast, not the nipple. So the small, flat nipple works just fine.

There are two situations, though, where you might encounter extra challenges. One is around day two or three when the amount of milk you are making rapidly increases and your breasts become very full and engorged. When this happens, flat nipples can seem to almost disappear into the curvature of the breast, and that can make it hard to get the baby latched on. The breast may be so engorged and firm that the baby can't get a mouthful into his mouth, and because he doesn't feel the nipple when he tries to latch on, he's not stimulated to start sucking (which would help release some of the milk). This problem becomes worse if you have intravenous fluids during labor, because some of those fluids you have taken in will also go to your breasts, and make them even fuller and firmer – sometimes painfully so.

Using Reverse Pressure Softening (as described on page 62) will help to move some of the fluid out of the tissues around the nipple, so the baby can latch on more effectively. You may also find it helps to hand express some milk and to rub your nipples to help them stand out as much as possible.

The other issue that sometimes crops up when women have small, flat nipples occurs when the baby has been given bottles, especially if he is given a bottle before he breastfeeds for the first time. You can see why: The baby who is just learning and figuring out this whole "where to get food" thing quickly learns to expect a large, firm, plastic nipple in his mouth and may have trouble latching on to the breast with a smaller flat nipple. You can put him in the position and encourage him to take your nipple into his mouth, but he may not suck because he's expecting to feel the pressure of a bottle nipple against his tongue and palate, and he doesn't understand that this kind of nipple will also give him milk.

The best strategy here is prevention. If your baby does need supplementation in the early weeks, giving that extra milk with a spoon, syringe, or (best of all) a lactation aid at the breast will help avoid this problem.

If your baby has been given bottles and you run into this problem, it can help to express a little milk just before you latch the baby on, so there are drops on the nipple. Just tasting the milk might encourage the baby to suck! Or you can squeeze your breast when the baby takes the nipple in his mouth, so he gets a little squirt of milk.

If that doesn't work, try having your baby self-attach. See page 51 for more information on this. Some mothers find it helps to take a bath with the baby to encourage self-attachment, maybe because everyone is feeling warm and relaxed in that situation. (Have a towel on the floor beside the tub to put your baby on when you get in or out of the tub – or do this when your partner is handy to pass the baby to you and retrieve him when you're done.)

Large Nipples

Women with very large, firm nipples can also sometimes run into difficulties, especially if the baby is relatively small at birth. That's because small babies often have small mouths! If the baby's mouth is really tiny, he may have trouble taking the entire nipple into his mouth and reaching the milk-containing ducts (which are normally in the breast tissue, behind the nipple) in order to compress them and encourage the flow of milk. Lactation consultants have nicknamed this "oroboobular disproportion."

Some women with large nipples find that they have "compressible" milk ducts within the nipple, so that if the baby can get most of the nipple into his mouth, breastfeeding will work fine. Some mothers have discovered that if the baby can get the nipple in his mouth, but not reach the milk ducts, the mother can compress her breast when the baby is sucking (like hand-expressing milk right into the baby), and he'll get the milk he needs.

In other cases, the nipple is just too big for the newborn baby to take into his mouth. Sometimes the mother's nipples are very firm and fibrous as well, and that can make it even harder for the baby to latch on or get any milk.

The good news about this situation is that it will resolve over time. Usually within a few weeks, the baby grows big enough to latch on well to even the largest nipples. The challenge is for the mother to keep up her milk supply (by frequent pumping and/or hand expression) and to find an alternate way to feed the baby. If the baby can latch on at all, using a lactation aid or compression to help the baby get milk may be the best plan. If he can't, the mother can pump or hand-express her milk and give it to the baby in whatever way is easiest for her. Even if she needs to give bottles, the baby will usually learn to take the breast when he's a bit bigger. (These large, firm nipples are a bit closer in size and consistency to bottle nipples, so the transition back to the breast is often a little easier than for mothers with smaller and flatter nipples.)

Inverted Nipples

Maybe your nipples are not just flat, but actually sink back into your breast, rather than protruding out. (You may have one nipple that sinks in, while the other one protrudes. That's not unusual.) Are you going to have a tough time breastfeeding? Probably not. Remember that the baby latches onto your breast, not just your nipple, so in most cases the baby will do just fine.

Try this little test: put your thumb on the areola (the darker circle of skin around your nipple) above the nipple, and your forefinger on the areola below the nipple. Now squeeze them together, pushing back slightly towards your ribcage at the same time. What happens? Did your nipple pop out? If so, you have what is sometimes called a "shy nipple."

Shy nipples are rarely a problem for breastfeeding mothers. Often mothers find that by the end of the pregnancy, they are protruding most of the time. If not, you can often get the nipple to come out just by applying some pressure as the baby prepares to latch on. You can also use a breast pump briefly before each feeding, or a "nipple everter," which is a syringe with the needle removed and the bottom end cut off and smoothed (you can just sand it down with a nail file). There are commercial nipple everters on the market, too. Once your baby gets a little practice, he'll be able to latch on, even if the nipple is inverted, and will pull the nipple out with his first couple of sucks.

What about the nipple that doesn't protrude at all when pressure is applied, or emerges briefly, then inverts again as soon as the pressure is released, or seems to become more inverted in response to pressure? In many cases, using a pump briefly before feeding may help to bring the nipple out, so the baby finds it easier to latch on. Some women have a lot of adhesions holding the nipple in the inverted position, and the milk-making ducts may also be constricted or closed up by these adhesions, so that breastfeeding is more problematic. If you find that your inverted nipples don't come out at all when you use a pump or apply pressure, you might want to talk to a Lactation Consultant or another breastfeeding expert before you have your baby.

In the past, women sometimes used breast shells to encourage inverted nipples to protrude. These shells are not the same as nipple shields (which look like thin bottle nipples). Breast shells come in two parts. The bottom part is like a flat doughnut, and the top like a dome; they are usually made of clear plastic. To wear them, you put your nipple through the hole in the middle of the doughnut part, attach the dome part on top, so the nipple is protected, and put a bra on top of the whole thing. The idea was that the pressure around the areola would force the nipple out and break down any adhesions. However, research has shown that this does not actually help – in fact, in at least one study (Alexander, Grant, & Campbell, 1992), the women who used the shells were more likely to stop breastfeeding early because of problems.

Pierced Nipples or Nipple Surgery

Your nipples may have been pierced many years ago or quite recently, or you may have more than one piercing; whatever the situation, you might be worried about how this will affect breastfeeding. Or perhaps you had surgery involving your nipples because of health issues or breast reductions or enhancements, and you've heard conflicting information about whether breastfeeding will be possible for you.

Pierced nipples are sometimes challenging for the breastfeeding mom, and sometimes not. Much depends on how the piercing was done, if ducts were damaged or blocked, if any infections developed, and how much scarring is present. Smaller piercings, obviously, are less likely to do as much damage.

Women vary quite a bit in how many duct openings they have in their nipples. Some have only three or four; some have as many as 12 or 13. Clearly, if you only have a small number and half of these are scarred over during the piercing, breastfeeding is more likely to be difficult.

Want some idea of what is going on? You can try hand-expressing colostrum towards the end of your pregnancy. You'll be able to see how many openings you have and how the milk is flowing. If you aren't making colostrum, or aren't making much, don't worry – for some women, their breasts really don't get started until just before the baby arrives. But if you do have some milk during pregnancy, that can be reassuring and encouraging!

If you are concerned about how piercings might affect breastfeeding, it can be helpful to remove any jewelry in the nipple while you are pregnant. There is considerable growth of ducts during each pregnancy, so if the jewelry isn't there, the ducts may repair themselves or you may grow new ducts in that area to transport milk. The earlier in pregnancy you are able to do this, the better.

If you do keep the jewelry in place, be sure to remove it when you are actually breastfeeding.

Nipple surgery is another area where the outcomes vary. Surgery done to treat an infected area may still leave most of the ducts intact. The surgery most likely to cause breastfeeding problems involves separating the nipple and areola from the breast and moving it to a new position. Often in doing this procedure, the surgeon makes an incision around the outside of the areola, in a circle around the nipple. This operation not only severs the milk ducts, but cuts through the nerves connected to the nipple. The nipples afterwards often feel quite insensitive to touch, and that can contribute to the problem, even if the ducts have partially regrown, because the sensation of the baby suckling is what normally causes the milk to be released by the mother. With that sensitivity gone or at least significantly reduced, it may be challenging to get the milk flowing.

When surgery to the nipple needs to be done, the ideal way to cut through the tissue is in a straight line radiating out from the nipple towards the mother's chest wall. This is likely to cut through the fewest number of milk-transporting ducts. If this is how your surgery was done, the odds are in your favor.

Another reason for nipple surgery is to change inverted nipples – especially the type that don't evert or protrude even when pressure is applied – to protruding nipples. This surgery often does a lot of damage to any milk ducts. Of course, in some cases of very inverted nipples, the milk ducts are already blocked or constricted, and the mother might have had difficulty with breastfeeding anyway.

What can you do if you've had surgery involving your nipples, or piercings, and you're just not sure how much breastfeeding will be affected? Many women who have had surgery to their nipples do breastfeed successfully. The first step is to make sure you get the help you need to get off to a good start. You'll want to carefully look at the chapters that follow so you will be prepared. You'll also want to consider your options for supplementing, in case that proves necessary.

Many women who have had some surgery or piercings and have low milk production with a first baby find that they have plenty of milk with a second or third baby. That's because more ducts grow during each pregnancy. There's also some evidence that breastfeeding one baby (even if you have to supplement as well) promotes duct growth, too – it's like a gift that your first baby gives to your next baby: extra milk!

Extra Nipples

Some women have extra nipples on the sides of their breasts, near their underarms, or below the breasts. They are all on what is called "the milk line" that runs from under the arm to your groin. (Think of a dog or cat, with two lines of nipples from front legs to back legs.) If you have extra nipples, they will always be on this line. You might just have one on one side, or you might have these auxiliary or supernumerary nipples on both sides.

In some cases, there is a fair amount of breast tissue present as well. In others, there is just a tiny nipple.

If you don't have much tissue there, you may not even notice the extra nipples – or may assume they are just moles or birthmarks – until you get pregnant. Just as your breasts get bigger (and more tender) thanks to the hormonal changes, so will these auxiliary nipples. They may enlarge and become darker in color. When you start producing milk, you may find that these smaller nipples will also leak milk. If you have more breast tissue around the nipple, it may become engorged and uncomfortable.

Because your baby won't be feeding on these extra nipples, any milk production will quickly shut down. If the area does become engorged to the point of being uncomfortable, you can try putting washed and lightly crushed cabbage leaves over the nipple and surrounding extra breast tissue; hold the leaves in place with a snug tank top. A cold pack on the area can also help. Research suggests both approaches can help (Mangesi & Dowswell, 2010; Arora, Vatsa, & Dadhwal, 2008; Nikodem, Danziger, Gebka, Gulmezoglu, & Hofmeyr, 1993).

Breasts

Remember when you hit puberty and your breasts started to grow? Typically, you start off with a firm "button" under the nipple, then you grow the small cone-shaped breasts seen in the early teen years. As you mature, your breasts normally become more rounded in shape, and this tends to increase during pregnancy. Of course, there are many variations.

However, some women find that their breasts don't develop as expected, and this can have implications for breastfeeding. While everyone's breasts are unique, there are some characteristics that can suggest breasts have developed in a way that isn't helpful for breastfeeding.

One Breast Much Smaller Than the Other

Yes, most women have breasts of slightly different sizes, but for some women, one breast is much smaller than the other – sometimes as much as two or three cups sizes smaller, and often a different shape as well (more cone-shaped or tubular than rounded). If this describes you, should you worry? Well, sometimes this difference shows that one breast developed normally, and one didn't. The smaller, less-developed breast might catch up (or at least get fuller) during pregnancy. If it doesn't, though, it may not produce much milk.

Is that a problem? Usually no. Most women can produce plenty of milk for one baby with only one breast doing all the work. You may get at least some milk from the smaller breast, but you may find your baby much prefers the breast that makes more (babies are greedy that way...). The baby may be willing to nurse for comfort on the second breast, after filling up on the first one.

If you have twins or triplets, though, or if your milk production is not as high as you'd like in the larger breast, you may need to supplement.

If your breasts are different sizes, but you're not quite sure if this means one is under-developed, it's worth checking with a knowledgeable Lactation Consultant or doctor who can help you figure out what's going on.

Under-Developed Breasts

Perhaps your breasts have always looked small and conical in shape, rather than rounded, and even during pregnancy this hasn't changed much. Usually your nipples and areolas are pale in color as well. These may be breasts that didn't fully develop at puberty, and you may not see many changes during pregnancy. You may find that you can produce enough milk, but need to feed your baby very frequently because you don't have much milk storage capacity (see page 22), or you may find that your milk supply is lower than your baby needs and supplementation is required.

This is not the same as having small breasts – if you have small breasts that are rounded in shape and increase somewhat in size during pregnancy, you will probably produce plenty of milk for your baby.

Tubular, Widely-Spaced Breasts

Maybe your breasts are about the same size, but they are shaped a little differently from the average breasts. Instead of being rounded, they are more cylindrical or tubular – the same width at the top (near your chest wall) as at the bottom (near your nipple). As well, they are widely spaced – often you can fit your whole hand in between them (and getting any cleavage in low-cut tops is pretty much impossible!). These breasts, too, may not be able to produce a full milk supply, as this somewhat unusual shape seems to indicate that the milk-producing ducts have not developed normally and supplementation may be needed.

Puffy or Notched Areolas

Sometimes the tubular breasts described above will have areolas that are puffy or have an indented edge where they meet the rest of the breast. Usually, the only difference between the areolas and the rest of the breast is a change in color. This can also be a sign of some unusual developmental features that can affect milk production.

Having one, or even more than one, of these variations doesn't mean you won't be able to breastfeed, or that you won't be able to breastfeed exclusively. I've known women with all of these breast and nipple variations who breastfed their babies; some even had an oversupply of milk! Breastfeeding is so vital to the health and survival of the human race that our bodies have all kinds of back-up systems to make it work despite anatomical problems.

But seeing some mothers producing an abundant milk supply definitely doesn't mean it will be that easy for every mother who has, for example, widely-spaced, tubular breasts. It can help to line up your breastfeeding support in advance, so that you'll have help to get things off to a good start, practical support at home in case you find yourself spending hours working on breastfeeding, and any equipment you might need to make this work (such as a supplementer you can use at the breast or a breast pump).

Breast Surgery

There have been entire books written on how breast surgery can affect breastfeeding, and there's at least one (excellent) website devoted to the topic: www.bfar.org. Not only does the site have practical information, it can put you in touch with a community of other mothers who can help you figure out solutions – because they've had the same challenges. This section can't duplicate all that, but here's an overview.

The most common types of breast surgeries are breast enhancements and breast reductions, followed by surgeries done for medical reasons, such as breast abscesses, biopsies, etc.

Breast enhancements often have minimal effect on breastfeeding. The surgeon basically creates a pocket in the breast to insert the implant, which is like a plastic bag usually filled with either saline or silicone. This can be done without causing a lot of damage to the milk ducts, and today many surgeons make an effort to avoid those ducts when possible.

However, some women who've had breast enhancement surgery do have difficulties with producing a full milk supply. It may be that the milk ducts were damaged or the nerves that transmit the sensations from the nipple to the brain were cut. But often it's the underlying reason for the surgery that is part of the problem. If you had breast enhancement done because your breasts always seemed small and under-developed, for example, you might not have had enough breast tissue for full lactation to begin with. Or perhaps you had the surgery in order to make your breasts match because one was much smaller than the other – and, as you will have seen in the section above, that may mean that breast was undeveloped.

Breast reductions are more likely to have a significant effect on breastfeeding because the surgery often involves cutting and removing more tissue, especially if the nipple is to be re-positioned. Milk ducts may be severed during this process, and the nerves which transmit sensations (and signal the breasts to release milk) may also be cut or damaged.

Because there is greater awareness of the importance of breastfeeding today, more surgeons are making an effort to do the surgery in a way that minimizes damage to the ducts and nerves involved.

Despite these concerns, many women who have had breast reduction surgery do breastfeed successfully. During pregnancy, the system of milk ducts grows and often will simply bypass any that have been cut or damaged by the surgery. Some women who find they don't have enough milk to completely supply their first baby born post-surgery will have lots of milk for their second and third babies, because more ducts re-grow during each pregnancy and breastfeeding experience.

Women do seem to have more milk if there has been a longer time between the surgery and the arrival of the baby.

If you've had breast surgery, your best strategy is to make sure you have help to get you off to the best possible start. You want to maximize milk production right from the beginning and be sure your baby is latched on and feeding well. By monitoring your baby's feeding and weight gain, you can determine whether supplementation is needed.

Large Breasts

You'd think that large breasts might give you an advantage – maybe more milk storage capacity or a bigger milk supply.

To a certain extent, that's true. Women with larger breasts do tend to have a somewhat larger milk storage capacity. However, research suggests that these women are less likely to breastfeed and less likely to continue breastfeeding if they start (Mok et al., 2008).

Why? There seems to be two main reasons. One is that it can be trickier to get the baby positioned and latched on if you have very large breasts. The second is that women often feel embarrassed about their more substantial breasts and feel they attract unwanted attention if they breastfeed in public. Often they get into a pattern of always giving bottles when they are out, and this can easily lead to early weaning.

If your breasts are a DD-cup or above, be aware that you may need extra help to get started with breastfeeding (Australian Breastfeeding Association, 2012). You may need to use different positions, such as the football hold (where you hold the baby at your side and underneath your breast). Lying on your side often works well because you don't have to support the baby and can use both hands to help with positioning. Women with larger, soft breasts sometimes find that the laid-back position doesn't work well for them because the baby "smooshes" into the breast.

Some women have found it helpful to use a sling (a triangular piece of fabric folded to make a straight strip and tied at the back of your neck, with the thicker piece of fabric under your breast) for the breast they are feeding the baby on. This helps to support the breast, so you can position the baby.

One strategy for breastfeeding in public without feeling you've exposed yourself to the world is to wear two bras. Yes, I know that sounds weird, but wait – there's an explanation. The top bra should be a nursing bra that fits you well. Underneath it, wear a regular, well-fitting bra (perhaps a sports bra) that you have cut two holes in, so that your nipple and areola fit through each hole. Now when you want to nurse your baby and you undo the flap of your nursing bra, your entire breast isn't exposed – just enough for the baby to latch on. The extra support from the two bras helps keep your breast where the baby can latch more easily, too. If that doesn't work well for you, or you find you're uncomfortable, you can do something similar with a camisole or tank top in a color similar to your bra color. Put the tank top on, put your bra on top, and figure out where to cut the circles.

Past Performance

If this isn't your first baby, you may have a breastfeeding history that is worrying you. Maybe you had a lot of breast or nipple pain with your previous baby, or didn't make enough milk, or experienced mastitis or thrush. What does this mean for you this time around?

If you're concerned, it might be worth exploring what happened with a La Leche League Leader, Lactation Consultant, or another breastfeeding expert. That person will be able to review all the circumstances, help you to figure out what went wrong, and perhaps give suggestions to prevent the problems this time.

I didn't have enough milk last time.

There are many possible reasons for this. It could be that you didn't get off to a good start – your baby didn't nurse frequently enough or effectively enough to establish good milk production. Or it could be that you had some of the developmental problems with your breasts discussed in this chapter.

Either way, the news is mostly good. During this pregnancy, those ducts will have grown and developed a bit more, so if your breasts were not adequately developed for full milk production last time, they may be now. While you may still not produce a full milk supply, you will probably need less supplementation. And if the problem was infrequent or ineffective feedings, you can get some help this time (or change your approach to baby care) to ensure that doesn't happen again.

My nipples were painfully sore.

Okay, you probably hate hearing "breastfeeding isn't supposed to hurt." But it's true. Pain in breastfeeding usually indicates that there is a problem, and the most common cause is that the baby is not latched on well. (We'll go into this in more detail in Chapter 5.) Don't take this as a criticism of you, your mothering, or your breastfeeding skills – the intended message is that there are usually solutions that can make breastfeeding more comfortable for you. So if it hurts, ask for help! You don't have to just suffer through this! It may not be related to the baby's positioning at the breast – sometimes babies have anatomical problems that make it impossible for them to latch and suck well. Or you may have a condition known as Reynaud's Phenomenon that causes your nipples to turn white after nursing and throb with pain, or you may have a yeast infection on your nipples (also called thrush), or a bacterial infection, or you may have a nipple "bleb" that blocks one of the milk ducts.

With all these different possible causes for nipple pain, there are obviously many possible solutions, so it's worth consulting an expert to help you figure out what's right for you and your situation. Get that help and you may be able to have a completely comfortable breastfeeding experience this time around.

I had mastitis and was very sick, so I had to wean.

Mastitis is an inflammation of the breast, usually caused by a bacterial infection. It can start off as a plugged duct or may appear quite suddenly, without the mother noticing any plugged ducts beforehand. Usually, part of your breast is red and inflamed-looking (although sometimes the infected area is deep in the breast, so you don't see any redness) and feels very tender. You often have a fever and achiness, and may feel nauseated as well.

Weaning is not recommended for mastitis. In fact, weaning can make it worse. It won't hurt your baby to drink your milk while you are sick with this condition, and the medications usually prescribed for mastitis are safe for your nursing baby.

If you wanted to breastfeed your previous baby or babies and ran into a lot of difficulties, it can be scary and stressful to be thinking about breastfeeding again. You can't help but anticipate that things will all go wrong. You might find the book *Breastfeeding Takes Two* by Stephanie Casemore helpful. The author helps mothers understand and deal with the challenges of coming to terms with a disappointing breastfeeding experience and creating a more positive experience the second time around.

What You Can Do Now

1. Time to take a good look at your breasts! Do yours have any of the potentially concerning characteristics described in this section? If so, think about what you might want to do to prepare for getting extra help: contacting (or at least getting contact information for) breastfeeding experts, purchasing some equipment, such as a feeding tube for supplementing if you think that would be needed, etc.

2. If you do have one or more special situations, check out some of the books that go into more detail about the issues you might be facing:

- *Defining Your Own Success* by Diana West (breastfeeding after breast surgery)

- *Making More Milk* by Diana West and Lisa Marasco (how to increase your milk production in a variety of challenging situations)

- *Breastfeeding Takes Two* by Stephanie Casemore (breastfeeding a second baby when it didn't go well with the first)

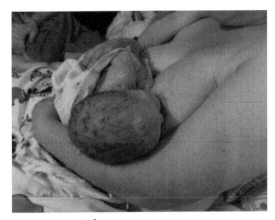

Chapter 4.
Birth Plans and
Breastfeeding Plans

There's a lot to decide when having a baby: doctor or midwife; home or hospital; medications, inductions, and other interventions. Depending on where you live and the kind of pregnancy you are experiencing, you may not have much choice about where you give birth and who provides your care. If your pregnancy is high-risk, for example, you may need to have an obstetrician provide your care and give birth in a hospital with the facilities to manage any anticipated complications. Or you may be low-risk and still need to see an obstetrician simply because there are no family doctors or midwives attending births in your community. Or you might have chosen to give birth with an obstetrician in attendance because you see that as the safest alternative.

In the medium-sized town where I live, we have two active midwifery practices, and the midwives catch babies (or sometimes coach partners on how to catch them!) both at home and in the hospital. Some family doctors also attend births, and there are a small group of obstetricians who take primarily higher-risk patients, including referrals from the midwives and family doctors when needed. A birth center is opening next year in the nearby large city, where women can have their babies in a home-like setting, cared for by midwives, but with quick access to additional medical care if needed.

Having a variety of care providers available gives women more choices about their caregivers and place of birth.

But I don't have to look far to see communities where there are fewer choices. You may live in an area where there are no midwives and none of the doctors attend home births, or you may be in a remote town where you need to travel long distances for care.

So your own birth plan might depend on:

- Whether your pregnancy is low-risk or higher-risk.

- The availability of options, such as midwifery care, home birth, birthing centers, etc.

- How you feel about pain medication in labor.

- Any research you have done on interventions and alternatives.

- The support system available to you.

- How you feel about home birth and hospital birth.

And now I'd like to suggest adding one more element into the mix: how your plans and choices for birth will affect breastfeeding.

We often think of birth and breastfeeding as being entirely separate, but, of course, how you give birth affects you and your baby and can make a big difference in how breastfeeding goes.

Who Will Catch Your Baby?

Most babies in North America are caught by midwives, family doctors, or obstetricians. (Of course, a few are caught by taxi drivers, daddies, and others...) The research suggests that when women give birth with midwives, they are more likely to breastfeed and to breastfeed longer.

Why? Part of this may be that women who opt for midwifery care are more interested in breastfeeding and more motivated to work through any challenges. But there are some aspects of midwifery care that may be valuable in promoting breastfeeding success:

- Continuity of care. Women usually see the same midwife or small team of midwives during prenatal appointments, labor and birth, and the first six weeks after the baby is born. This means the midwife is aware of any issues that might affect breastfeeding, helping her to provide effective care. In other models, the mother may see one doctor (an obstetrician) during pregnancy and birth, and another (a pediatrician) once her baby is born – and the pediatrician might not be aware of problems the mother had that might be related to breastfeeding challenges.

- Time. Solving breastfeeding problems often takes time. Your helper needs to be able to observe the baby at the breast, discuss the history of the problem with you, and perhaps try a couple of different possible solutions. Midwives generally are able to schedule longer appointments with their clients and take the time to explore these issues.

- Minimizing interventions. Many midwives attend births at home; those who attend births in the hospital usually try to minimize interventions there, too.

- Community connections. Midwives are usually well connected to breastfeeding support groups in the community (such as La Leche League) and will encourage mothers to attend meetings or drop-in events, call volunteers for help, or email questions to hotlines. Research is very clear about the importance of this ongoing community support for breastfeeding success.

A family doctor may also offer continuity of care, looking after you before and after the birth, and your new baby once she is born. Doctors vary considerably in their intervention rates and expertise about breastfeeding, so it is worth asking some questions, just so you know what to expect.

Obstetricians focus on pregnancy and birth; pediatricians focus on the baby's health after he's born. This selective focus can be a good thing at times, but it's not always helpful for breastfeeding. The question is: Who should help if there is a breastfeeding problem, such as sore nipples? The obstetrician because they are the mother's nipples? Or the pediatrician because the soreness may be caused by the baby having a tongue-tie or other issue? And like other caregivers, obstetricians and pediatricians may be very helpful and supportive or may be generally uninterested.

In a study done in Ontario, Canada, the researchers found that simply visiting a doctor in the weeks after having a baby, for any reason (even if the problem was unrelated to breastfeeding), was a risk factor for weaning (Sheehan, Krueger, Watt, Sword, & Bridle, 2001). Seeing a midwife, however, was not.

If you are considering a caregiver, or wondering if you should change caregivers, or just want to know whether you can look forward to a lot of help and support from your doctor, here are some questions you might ask:

1. What percentage of the women you care for breastfeed their babies? What percentage are still breastfeeding exclusively at six months? Breastfeeding at 12 months? *(The answers to these questions should be as high as possible. Of course, the mothers are influenced by other factors as well, but within any community, you'll find that some caregivers have more breastfeeding mothers in their practices than others.)*

2. In what situations would you advise a woman to wean her baby? *(The answer to this question should be a very short list! A small number of medications and illnesses do require weaning, but other than that, most challenges and situations have solutions.)*

3. What do you generally suggest to a woman who has sore nipples? *(Some responses you DON'T want to hear are "wean, use a nipple shield, or pump and give milk in a bottle." What you are hoping for in response to this question is some awareness of the many possible causes of sore nipples, and some suggestion that the caregiver would either make a full evaluation of the situation or refer the mother to someone who can make that evaluation.)*

4. What breastfeeding support groups in the community do you suggest people get in touch with? *(Research has shown that connecting with a breastfeeding support group, like La Leche League, makes a big difference in how long a mother is able to breastfeed. A doctor or midwife who can provide you with a list of places – or even just one or two places – for breastfeeding support shows awareness of the research and solid connections in the community.)*

Where Will Your Baby Be Born?

Not surprisingly, perhaps, giving birth at home is linked with higher rates of breastfeeding success. The mother and baby are able to stay together 24/7 with minimal intervention or interference – a good setting for breastfeeding. If you are considering a home birth, add easier breastfeeding as another reason to give it a try.

But mothers planning hospital births can succeed, too.

If you have a choice, look for a hospital that is Baby-Friendly. The Baby-Friendly Hospital Initiative is a program that was initiated by the World Health Organization and UNICEF to protect the health of babies around the world. To qualify for the Baby-Friendly designation, a hospital has to meet ten guidelines.

They are:

1. Have a written breastfeeding policy that is routinely communicated to all healthcare staff.

2. Train all healthcare staff in skills necessary to implement this policy.

3. Inform all pregnant women about the benefits and management of breastfeeding.

4. Help mothers initiate breastfeeding within one half-hour of birth.

5. Show mothers how to breastfeed and maintain lactation, even if they should be separated from their infants.

6. Give newborn infants no food or drink other than breastmilk, not even sips of water, unless medically indicated.

7. Practice rooming in - that is, allow mothers and infants to remain together 24 hours a day.

8. Encourage breastfeeding on demand.

9. Give no artificial teats or pacifiers (also called dummies or soothers) to breastfeeding infants.

10. Foster the establishment of breastfeeding support groups and refer mothers to them on discharge from the hospital or clinic.

The program also restricts use by the hospital of free formula or other infant care aids (such as name cards on bassinets, etc.) provided by formula companies. Mothers who choose to feed their babies formula are not forgotten in this initiative. They receive one-to-one teaching on how to safely prepare and feed formula. This is important because research has shown that the majority of parents make mistakes in formula preparation, increasing the risks of infection and other illnesses. The goal of the initiative is to improve the health of all babies, not just those who are breastfed.

These ten steps are all based on research, and hospitals that implement them have more mothers starting out and continuing to breastfeed.

No Baby-Friendly hospitals available to you? Try to find out what you can about the routines in the hospital you are planning to use. If you meet new mothers through a group like La Leche League, you'll be able to find out if there are any particular challenges and learn what other women have done to help breastfeeding succeed despite potential setbacks.

Birth Interventions

While choosing the right caregiver and place of birth can make a big difference, what goes on during labor and birth also affects breastfeeding. Let's look at some of the common interventions in hospital births and how they might affect the baby.

Induction of Labor

Many physicians will recommend inducing labor for a variety of reasons: concerns that the baby is getting too big, trying to avoid holidays, the "due date" has gone by, etc. There are also significant medical concerns that may require induction, such as high blood pressure, diabetes, etc., but many inductions are elective.

If the induction is done with pitocin given intravenously, the mother will receive fluids throughout the induction process (which can last for many hours). Those IV fluids can cause problems in a couple of ways. First, the baby is born with extra fluid in his system. Then when he starts peeing those fluids out, it makes him look as though he has lost a lot of weight, and hospital staff may start recommending supplementation. Some researchers have suggested that the baby's weight at 24 or 36 hours should be used as the baseline instead, so that the extra fluid isn't "counted" in calculating weight loss (Noel-Weiss, Woodend, & Groll, 2011; Watson, Hodnett, Armson, Davies, & Watt-Watson, 2012).

Some of that fluid will go into the mother's breasts, usually arriving there around day two or three when her breasts are also filling up with milk. This edema will make her breasts painfully swollen, and it can be very difficult for the baby to latch on. Some babies won't be able to latch at all.

Even if the induction is not done with IV fluids, there is a risk that the baby will be born somewhat prematurely. His breastfeeding skills might not be fully developed, so he may struggle to latch on well, or he might get tired easily, falling asleep before he's had a full feeding. Even with the best testing available, miscalculations are sometimes made and babies are pushed out of the uterus too early. Letting your baby choose his own birthday (when possible) will help ensure he's ready to breastfeed effectively.

Intravenous Fluids

In some hospitals, IV fluids are routinely given when women arrive in labor. The idea is that by putting the IV in place right away, if medications are needed, they can be easily added, or if an emergency C-section is needed, the IV will already be in place, speeding up the process.

However, as mentioned above, the IV fluids can cause problems in two ways. Some fluid goes into the baby, so his weight at birth is higher than it would be otherwise, and when he gets rid of that fluid, he appears to have lost an excessive amount of weight. This may lead to pressure to supplement, and supplementing can cause many breastfeeding problems. In addition, some of the fluids go to the mother's breasts and cause edema just as she is engorged with milk. The added edema can make it very difficult for the baby to latch on and get milk effectively.

One way to avoid these problems, even if your hospital feels strongly about having an IV line in "just in case," is to ask for what is called a "hep lock" instead. This is where the needle is inserted into the vein and a small amount of heparin is added to prevent the blood in the vein from clotting and closing up the spot where the needle is inserted. The other end is then closed. If fluids or IV medication are needed, this can be quickly re-opened to connect with the tubing, and there is no fuss about getting the needle inserted.

Epidural Anesthetic

Epidural anesthetic for labor and birth has become increasingly popular over the years. In many places in North America, the majority of women will have epidurals during labor. It allows the woman in labor to be awake and aware of what is going on, while feeling no painful sensations, and it has minimal effect on the baby's breathing and activity level (compared to other medications). There are also fewer side effects for the mother than some of the medications used previously. Sounds ideal, doesn't it?

However, research has shown that epidurals can affect breastfeeding in several ways.

- Women getting epidurals must also get IV fluids, because one side-effect of the epidural is a drop in blood pressure that can be quite serious. So the mother who has an epidural is likely to have the IV-related problems described above.

- Another common side effect of an epidural is that the mother may develop a fever. When this happens, hospitals usually separate the mother and baby while tests are run to determine whether or not the mother has an infection that could harm her baby. Even if the mother tries to pump or hand-express milk during this separation, she may have some trouble establishing a good milk supply. If the baby is fed by bottle while they are separated, she may have difficulty getting him to breastfeed well once they are together again.

- Epidurals increase the risk of other interventions, such as forceps, vacuum extraction, and C-sections, all of which have their own set of added risks for breastfeeding. This is partly because epidurals increase the risk of the baby being in a difficult position for birth (such as face-up rather than face-down, etc.). It is also more difficult for a mother who has an epidural in place to push effectively.

- The medication in the epidural is passed along to the baby and can affect his ability to latch and suckle. One study measured the levels of medication in the umbilical cord; the researchers found that the longer the epidural is in place, the higher the level of medication in the cord (Loftus, Hill, & Cohen, 1995). And, of course, the cord transfers the medication to the baby. But does this affect the baby? Yes, according to research (Szabo, 2013). Babies whose mothers had epidurals in labor have more difficulty latching at the breast, are more likely to have an uncoordinated suck, and are more likely to be supplemented. Breastfeeding is a fairly complex activity, and the medication in the epidural seems to hinder the baby's ability to make it work. However, other studies have shown little difference in breastfeeding outcomes when mothers have epidurals; much depends on the level of breastfeeding help and support available in the hospital. In other words, the potential problems related to epidurals CAN be overcome if you get good help.

- The effects of the epidural on the baby may last for a few hours, a few days, or a few weeks, depending on the medication used and the length of time the epidural was in place.

There's a well-known video usually called "Delivery Self-Attachment" (the original is in Swedish), which shows how newborn babies, placed on their mother's abdomens and with little or no help from anyone, will move to the breast, find the nipple, and latch on. The video shows several babies doing this. Then a baby whose mother had an epidural is shown. This baby attempts to find the breast and nipple, but struggles and acts confused. When he gets to the nipple, he doesn't seem to know what to do with it. This is similar to the behavior many Lactation Consultants and La Leche League Leaders report with babies who have been exposed to epidural medications.

Other Pain Medications

Some other pain medications (such as meperidine/pethidine) given in labor can potentially depress the baby's breathing and make him too lethargic and sleepy to breastfeed well. The goal is usually to give these medications several hours before the baby is born, so the mother's body has time to clear the drugs. A newborn baby's system can take a long time to get rid of any medication that is present.

Of course, that's challenging for a couple of reasons. One, the time when a mother is most likely to want pain medication is towards the end of her labor, since the contractions get more intense as time goes on. And two, it can be very hard to look at a woman in labor and accurately predict how much longer it will take before her baby is born. Sometimes women who have taken 15 hours to get to five cm. dilation will speed up significantly at that point and be ready to push the baby out an hour or two later.

Forceps and Vacuum Extractors

Sometimes when a mother's cervix is fully dilated, the baby still seems not to be coming quickly enough. This can be because the baby is not in a good position for being born, or because the mother is having difficulty pushing effectively (the risk of both of these is increased by the use of epidural anesthetic). Then a doctor may use either forceps or a vacuum extractor to help pull the baby out through the birth canal.

Many babies who have had this kind of birth intervention will have bruising or a hematoma on their heads, and they often behave as though they have headaches. Just holding them in the usual breastfeeding position may cause distress and resistance.

C-Sections

About one-third of mothers in the U.S., and between one-quarter and one-third of mothers in Canada, will have surgery for the birth of their babies. Some will be planned and some will take place after labor is underway.

Research has shown that mothers who have Caesarean sections are less likely to breastfeed and are more likely to wean early, even if they start (Karlstrom, Lindgren, & Hildingsson, 2013). The C-section birth includes interventions we already know can cause problems (IV fluids, epidurals), plus new ones: The mother needs to recover from major surgery and may be exhausted and sore; the surgical incision may make it difficult to find a comfortable position for breastfeeding; hospital policies may separate mother and baby during the first few hours and delay the start of breastfeeding; and the mother is at risk of infection and other problems which may separate her from her baby for a longer period of time.

Episiotomy

An episiotomy is an incision made in the tissue at the bottom of your vagina, to widen it and make it easier for the baby to come out. Some doctors feel that this prevents tearing (although the logic of a cut to prevent a tear seems...not very logical) and find the straight cut easier to sew up, so they perform episiotomies fairly routinely. Others reserve it for situations where the baby needs to be born quickly because it is in distress, or when forceps are needed to help the baby out.

An episiotomy usually is cut through both skin and muscle, and can be very painful as it heals. Some become infected, causing more pain. An episiotomy can make it more difficult to find a comfortable position for breastfeeding, especially if the mother wants to sit up or semi-recline. Extra pillows can help – a pillow under your knees if you are semi-reclined or between your knees if you are lying on your side may reduce the tension on the stitches. And take extra care in keeping the area clean to reduce the risk of infection.

Cutting the Cord

The umbilical cord, which has connected the baby to the placenta during the pregnancy, is normally cut soon after the birth. (Some women will choose what is called a "lotus birth" where the cord is not cut, but remains attached to both baby and placenta until it dries up on its own and falls off. The placenta is kept wrapped in plastic bag and moved with the baby as needed.)

Some caregivers will cut the cord as soon as the baby is born. This reduces the amount of blood the baby gets from the cord, which can mean he has lower iron stores and is at greater risk of becoming anemic.

Letting the cord finish pulsating on its own maximizes the amount of blood the baby gets, increasing his iron stores. Iron is an important nutrient for babies for overall health, brain development, etc. However, this extra blood means that the baby is also at higher risk of developing jaundice, a common concern for newborns and a common reason for supplementation (often unnecessary).

Deep Suctioning

Before a baby is born, his uninflated lungs are filled with mucous and amniotic fluid. That's normal. The birth process is designed to squeeze out much of that mucous and fluid as the baby emerges from the birth canal and is lifted up to his mother's arms. Sometimes, though, babies have a lot of mucous and need some help in clearing it. Your doctor or midwife can use a suction bulb to pull out the excess mucous, making it easier for the baby to breathe.

Sometimes a baby who is feeling stressed in utero will have a bowel movement before he is born. This turns the amniotic fluid greenish in color and becomes a problem if the baby breathes in some of this contaminated fluid. If your doctor or midwife sees that there is meconium (the name for the baby's first poops) in the fluid, he or she will want to suction the baby to remove as much as possible. If the meconium gets into the baby's lungs, it can cause pneumonia.

Some doctors will do fairly vigorous or deep suctioning of the baby routinely, just in case of problems with mucous or meconium. This can be very stressful for the newborn – the tissues of the mouth and throat are sensitive – and may make him resist breastfeeding. His thinking is that last time something went into his mouth, it hurt and was scary! So he's keeping his mouth clamped shut now, thank you very much!

Making Your Choices

I want to be really clear: I am not saying women should not have epidurals, pain medication in labor, C-sections, etc. All of these available interventions are valuable and can reduce or eliminate pain, and even save lives. I believe women should be able to choose the labor and birth that is right for them (given, of course, that you need to be flexible to respond to any unexpected situations or complications that might arise).

I believe, though, that choices should be made with full information – and some of these interventions have the potential to make breastfeeding more challenging. That doesn't mean you shouldn't choose them if that's what you want. But you might also want to plan for extra breastfeeding help once your baby is born, or express some colostrum prenatally, so it will be available if your baby has some difficulties latching on at first, or plan to bring in some research on the effects of IV fluids on newborn weight loss in case you get pressure to supplement, etc.

Delaying the First Feeding

As we have discussed elsewhere, your new baby is born ready to begin breastfeeding and, if simply allowed to lie on your chest, will usually find the breast and latch on within an hour or so. This first feeding is important: It gives the baby the antibodies and immune factors needed to protect him from the germs he's now exposed to; it gives the baby nutrition to stabilize blood sugar and start the passing of meconium; and it starts up the milk-producing system for the mother and helps contract the mother's uterus to prevent excessive bleeding. Wait too long and the baby may become sleepy and breastfeeding will be harder. The photo below shows a baby nursing within the first hour after birth.

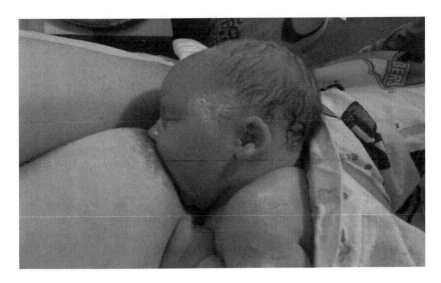

However, some hospitals have policies or procedures that require prompt separation of mother and baby. They may require that the baby be examined in an isolette with an overhead heat lamp, and then they may take the baby away to be weighed and bathed. A few places still have newborn nurseries where the babies are taken, so the mother can get some rest.

Keeping mothers and babies together, so the babies can breastfeed frequently, is very important for establishing good milk production, though. If this isn't possible, you may want to begin hand-expressing your milk as soon as you can to get the process going.

Overcoming Early Challenges

The best-laid plans don't always work out. Perhaps you were hoping for an unmedicated birth at home, but ended up having your labor induced, getting an epidural, and finally a Caesarean section. Your baby was scooted off to the nursery and was sleepy and reluctant to breastfeed by the time you saw her. You couldn't get her to latch on at all. The nurse said they'll have to give her a bottle of formula to keep her blood sugar up.

You can see your dreams of breastfeeding slipping away. What can you do?

Keep in mind all the things you've learned about how breastfeeding works and what you can do to protect it:

- Begin hand-expressing your milk as soon as possible. Ask for someone who can teach you if you find it difficult. (Hand-expression is far more effective in the first few days before the milk volume increases). Express the milk into sterile containers and ask that this be used if any supplementation is needed. Aim to express every two to three hours, including during the night.

- Keep your baby skin-to-skin as much as possible. This reduces stress and helps maintain a healthy blood sugar level, *even if the baby doesn't feed*.

- Try different positions for breastfeeding to see if your baby responds better to one.

- If you need to supplement, use something other than a bottle. In the first few days, the baby only needs small amounts of colostrum – his tummy is the size of a chickpea! Use a small spoon to give him the milk you have expressed.

- Once your milk volume increases, if the baby is still not latching on, you can start using a pump. There may come a point where you decide to give your pumped milk with a bottle rather than a spoon, syringe, or cup. If you maintain a good milk supply, you will usually be able to get the baby to the breast eventually, even if it takes a few weeks. Maximize the amount of skin-to-skin time.

- Be patient with your baby and with yourself. It can take time for the medications from labor and birth to wear off. Some researchers have found effects from certain drugs in the baby up to four weeks after the birth.

- Seek help early on. If your baby hasn't started to breastfeed or is not breastfeeding well (you have sore nipples, the baby is not gaining well, etc.) get in touch with a Lactation Consultant or La Leche League Leader for more information and guidance.

Labor interventions can make breastfeeding more difficult. But with good help, these difficulties can be overcome.

Planning to Breastfeed

Let's do a little math. In the beginning, babies often nurse for 30 to 40 minutes, or longer, at each feeding. Feedings are often about two hours apart, counting from the beginning of the previous feeding.

That means you can easily spend 40 minutes times 12 or SIX HOURS a day breastfeeding. Later, this will be easier: Feedings will be shorter, you'll be able to do other things while breastfeeding, and you'll have figured out a rough routine. But in the beginning, it can be pretty overwhelming. Let's face it, you probably don't have six spare hours in your day. Some other tasks are going to have to be dropped or minimized.

So while you are making birth plans and preparing for the birth experience, it can help to think ahead and plan to make those early weeks when you are learning to breastfeed a bit easier.

Meals

You need to eat. You're recovering from birth and making milk for your baby. But who has time to cook? Not you!

- During pregnancy, consider making extra meals and stocking your freezer. There are many great ideas for make-ahead meals on the internet – just search for ones that appeal to you.

- One mother expecting twins hired a personal chef for a day. She discussed her food preferences with him. He created a list of meals, went shopping, prepped the food in her own kitchen, and filled her freezer with tasty, delicious dishes that kept the family going for several weeks. And she says it cost her much less than eating out would have.

- If your family or friends are interested in having a baby shower for you, maybe they'll consider making it a food shower as well. Each guest could bring something for your freezer, as well as a baby item.

- No time to prep food in advance? There are stores where all the prep work has been done – you simply go in, make up the meals you want, and pay for them. Regular grocery stores often have lots of ready-to-go meals – add a salad and fruit and you're done.

- Ordering in food? Try to balance the typical fast food meals with salads, fruit, and healthy drinks (water's good!). You'll feel better and you are already teaching your baby about what foods he should eat when he starts on solids. (It's true: The flavors come through in your milk, and mothers who eat plenty of veggies while breastfeeding have babies who choose veggies more often when they are older.)

Housework

When people offer to get you baby gifts, consider putting "maid service" on the list. Someone to come in and clean for a few weeks after the birth might make a big difference in how you feel.

Once the baby is born, keep a running list of things to be done. If a visitor drops by and says casually, "Let me know if there is anything I can do" – you can hand over the list and encourage them to pick something (like throwing in a load of laundry or vacuuming the living room).

Taking Care of Yourself

Inevitably, taking care of your new baby will come first. That's natural. But you need to figure out ways to take care of your needs, too. You are recovering from pregnancy (a major event in your life), birth, possibly surgery (if you had a C-section), and are now taking on the challenging task of nurturing a new baby.

Talk to your partner about what things will help you stay healthy, both physically and emotionally.

- Consider scheduling a weekly massage for the first few weeks after your baby is born. Your body will be changing and your muscles may ache from carrying the baby and sitting up to breastfeed. A massage will help you feel better and sleep better.

- Does your diet need some fine-tuning? Maybe some green smoothies, more salads, or other small changes will help you with your recovery. Many experts recommend Vitamin D supplements and omega-3 supplements to help you feel better not just physically, but mentally as well.

- You may not feel much like exercising at first, but even a daily walk around the block (just pop the baby into a sling or carrier) will be good for you and your baby. See if your community offers postpartum yoga classes or mom and baby swim groups and sign up now!

- Many new mothers feel isolated and lonely. Groups like La Leche League and other organizations for new mothers give you somewhere to go with your baby and opportunities to meet other new moms. You can start attending La Leche League while you are pregnant; some other groups require you to wait until your baby is born. Check out the options in your community.

Equipment for Breastfeeding

You can't avoid the ads. Every parenting magazine or website says you need a breast pump, breast pads, a super-duper nursing bra, breastfeeding pillows, lotions for sore nipples, teas to increase milk production, nipple shields to protect your nipples, etc., etc., etc.

Truth is, you have everything you need: breasts and (soon) a baby. Done.

Of course, those other items can be helpful in certain situations. If your baby is born so prematurely that he can't breastfeed, a pump may help you establish a milk supply and get milk for him. If you need to go back to work while your baby is small, a pump can allow you to provide milk for your baby while you're away. Breastfeeding pillows sometimes make positioning easier, but sometimes cause problems. Nipple shields are occasionally useful, but more often lead to decreasing milk production and breastfeeding difficulties.

And what about bras? Most women see their breasts increase by one cup size when they are breastfeeding (not counting the more dramatic increase in size at day three or four). But there's some variation in that, so don't go overboard buying bras while you are still pregnant – get one or two to get you through the first couple of weeks, then plan to buy more.

Some women don't use nursing bras at all – they are more comfortable with stretchy sports bras and just pull the entire cup down to nurse the baby. If you do use a nursing bra, try to find one where you can undo the nursing flap with one hand (the other will be busy holding the baby). Avoid underwire bras, which can put pressure on the ducts and cause problems. If you are smaller-breasted, you may be able to skip wearing a bra and just wear a camisole or tank top.

So what do you need to buy now? Not much: a bra or two for those early weeks, perhaps a pump if you know you'll be back to work early. The rest can wait until you see if it's something you actually need. With luck, you, your breasts, and your baby will do just fine on your own.

What You Can Do Now

1. With your partner, create a birth plan. This isn't something that is set in stone, and you may not even share it with your caregivers. What you want is to be sure that you and your partner are on the same page when it comes to interventions and other plans, so that he or she can give you the support you need.

2. Find out what breastfeeding help is available in your community. If you are planning a hospital birth, does the hospital have IBCLCs (International Board Certified Lactation Consultants) on staff? Is there a breastfeeding clinic? Will a public health nurse with breastfeeding training come to your home to help you?

3. If you have not taken or signed up for prenatal classes, consider taking one – ideally one taught by a private educator who is not connected to the hospital. You'll learn about the possible interventions and hospital routines in detail, so you can make the choices that work for you. You'll also get techniques and strategies to help you manage pain in labor, helping you avoid some of the interventions.

4. Make sure you've taken breastfeeding into consideration in your plans for the postpartum time. Do you have some meals prepared in advance or have you taken other steps to free up time for breastfeeding? What plans can you make to be sure you have what you need to recover physically and emotionally? Can you sign up for postpartum yoga, mother and baby groups, massages, etc. now?

5. Think about the equipment you might need to help you breastfeed. Buying a bra or two for breastfeeding in advance is a good idea; you can get the rest later.

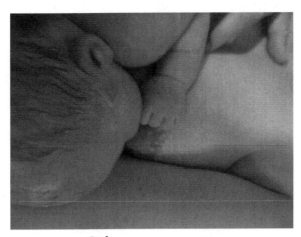

Chapter 5.
What Your Baby Knows About Breastfeeding

Most mothers imagine breastfeeding is something *they* do. They figure out when it's time to feed again, they bring the baby to the breast, they put the nipple in baby's mouth, they make sure the latch is good, and unlatch the baby when the feeding is done.

The truth is, your baby knows a lot more than most people think about breastfeeding. He's born with the instincts and skills to make breastfeeding work – just like other baby mammals are. (If you've ever seen a cat with newborn kittens or a baby calf with its mother, you'll know that they are clearly hard-wired to find food. Our babies are too.)

Of course, mothers also have built-in skills for breastfeeding, and those mesh nicely with the baby's. Human babies aren't as physically strong and capable as some others (that baby calf can walk and run within hours of birth – your baby won't be walking for year or so! That's a big difference!), so they need more help from their mothers. Mama cow just has to stand still while her baby latches on; you may need to do a bit more than that!

But maybe not as much as you think.

Holding Your Baby

If someone hands you a fussy baby, what do you do? Most women, without even thinking about it, will hold the baby vertically against their chests or shoulders, with baby's tummy against their chest, one hand behind baby's shoulders and the other behind his bottom. This natural position for soothing is also the perfect spot for the baby to begin feeding.

What typically happens is that the baby will first snuggle into your chest a little, and then will lift up his head, or even throw his head back. Sometimes parents think this is because the baby's neck muscles aren't very strong, or imagine it's just a random movement, but researchers who have observed many babies tell us that it's deliberate. It seems to be part of the way the baby orients himself: "Hmm, I am in contact with my mother's body, let's look around and see where I am – yup, there is her head, so those nice things with the milk in them should be a little lower, one on either side." The photo below shows a newborn at the breast.

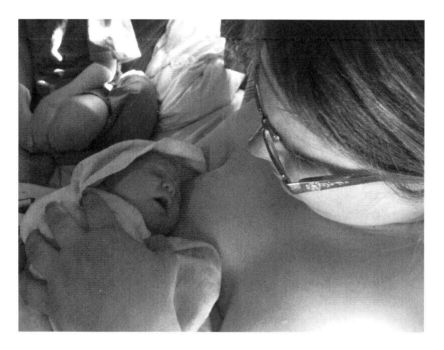

And, in fact, if your baby is hungry, what he'll do next is move to one side or the other, heading towards the breast. Some babies do this very vigorously – they practically throw themselves sideways. Others kind of squirm or shuffle to one side.

These natural movements towards the breast are more likely to happen if you and your baby are skin-to-skin – layers of clothes can be confusing, although many babies do manage to figure it out.

Some experts feel that when we pick up a crying newborn and hold him in what we think of as a breastfeeding position (horizontally across our tummies, head towards the breast) that we are actually confusing the baby. His instinctive expectations are to be held vertically, in that soothing position, so that he can find his own way to the breast. (Of course, an older, more experienced baby is less concerned – once they've mastered breastfeeding, they don't mind at all being moved into breastfeeding position right away.)

Latching On

In recent years, a lot of attention has been paid to how babies latch on to the breast. Nurses, Lactation Consultants, and others have used a variety of techniques to help mothers get their babies properly positioned and attached to the breast.

Some of this was necessary: Thirty years ago, breastfeeding rates were very low, and many new mothers had only seen babies being fed with bottles. So when they were given their babies to feed, they imitated bottle-feeding: The mother held her baby on his back, as if she was going to put a bottle in his mouth, and the baby had to turn his head sideways to try to latch on to the nipple. The mother was also used to seeing babies taking just the rubber nipple of the bottle into their mouths, so she expected her baby to latch on to just her nipple. This was a recipe for sore nipples and feeding problems (try lying on your back, then turning your head sideways to drink. Not easy!)

Mothers were encouraged to position the baby lying on his side, his tummy against her tummy, so he could latch on without turning his head. Definitely an improvement. But the baby still didn't always take the breast deep enough into his mouth, and soon nurses started using the "RAM" technique. RAM stood for Rapid Arm Movement, but it was very descriptive – as soon as the nurse saw the baby open his mouth to take the nipple, she'd quickly push his head onto the breast.

Sometimes this worked. But more often, it made babies mad. Imagine you were just about to take a drink, and someone suddenly pushed the back of your head. And then imagine that you also had a headache, as many babies do after difficult births – yeah, even worse.

Many babies would push back against the pressure of the hand, so they didn't latch at all. Others grabbed the nipple and didn't get a good deep latch.

More attempts were made to shape the breast and the nipple to help the baby get on well. Eventually, though, researchers and people who work with mothers and babies realized that babies know best. Given the right situation and opportunity, the baby would latch on and do so beautifully.

Today, most breastfeeding experts encourage mothers to start with what some call "laid-back breastfeeding." It's ideal for letting the baby show off his skills and abilities, and for getting breastfeeding off to a good start. There's more detailed information about this in the next chapter, but basically here's what you do:

- Get in a comfortable, semi-reclining position.

- Put the baby, tummy-down, on your chest.

- Let the baby find the breast and latch on. Help a little or a lot, as needed.

When the baby latches on in this position, he is coming down onto the nipple from above and will naturally get a good, deep latch, with the nipple well back in his mouth. In other positions, with the mother sitting upright, the baby is reaching up to the nipple, and it's easier to just latch on to the nipple, not the breast.

You don't have to use this position forever, but during the early days, it's ideal. It's comfortable and restful for you, your baby will latch on well, and you're working together to get breastfeeding going. The photo below shows laid-back positioning.

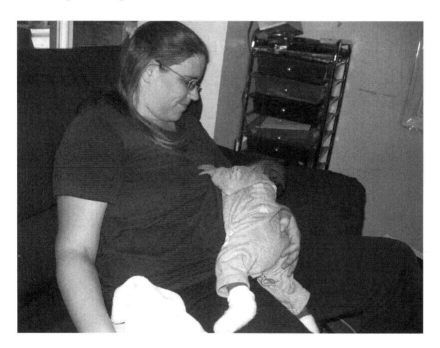

When to Feed

Your baby doesn't know the mechanics of milk production and how the breast functions, but he knows exactly how to establish a good milk supply, how to adjust the milk supply to meet his needs, and how to change the fat content and other components of the milk as his needs change over time. All we have to do is follow his lead.

One of the significant differences between formula and human milk is that formula is always the same (unless, of course, the manufacturer finds a cheaper type of oil to add to it, or changes the composition by adding some ingredient extracted from fungus), while human milk changes at every feeding. Sometimes it has more of a certain type of antibody, for example, or more fat.

Milk produced in the evening or night has components that help to relax the baby and encourage sleep. If the mother has eaten garlic or foods with other flavors, those flavors come through in the milk. We don't always understand the purpose of all these changes, but many of them are clearly important for the baby.

Typically, a newborn baby will nurse within the first hour after birth (although for some babies, medications or interventions in labor and birth, or health issues, may mean this needs to be delayed). This first feeding is important because it initiates milk production, helps reduce the mother's risk of bleeding, and starts the learning process. After that, many babies (especially if the birth has been challenging) will sleep or rest for a few hours. (Hint: Mom – you should rest, too!)

When the baby wakes up again, he often starts into what feels like a marathon of nursing. The books say you should expect "eight to 12 feedings in 24 hours." Your baby may have his own ideas about that. Some will nurse for short periods of time every half hour or so, usually with a couple of longer stretches, and some will nurse relatively infrequently. Those patterns often change as the baby grows.

The baby uses these feeding patterns to make sure the milk he gets is meeting his needs. Let's say he's going through a period of rapid brain growth, when he needs more of the fats in the milk to build brain cells. Frequent, short feedings will bring him more of the high-fat milk.

Or let's say it's a hot day and your baby needs more liquids. He may go a bit longer between feedings, and then want to switch quickly from one breast to the other, so he gets more of the lower-fat milk to quench his thirst.

Maybe there is a virus going around. You and your baby have both been exposed to it. As your baby starts to feel a bit ill, he nurses more often to maximize the antibodies and immune factors he will get from your milk to reduce the impact of the illness.

As a new nursing mother, there may be many times that you wonder, "Why is my baby nursing so often today?" or "Hmm, what's causing him to nurse less often this afternoon than usual?" Often there is no obvious answer. Trust that your baby knows what he's doing. He's adjusting the components of your milk and your milk production to meet his ever-changing needs. All you have to do is recognize his cues and feed him when he asks.

Frequency Days: Nobody really knows why these happen, and probably there are different reasons for them. One may be to increase milk production. If you were feeding your baby with bottles and found he was still hungry after each feeding, you could increase the amount of milk in the bottle. But the breastfeeding baby who wants more milk can't just email you a note requesting an increase. To get more milk produced, he needs to nurse more often for a couple of days to send the message to the milk ducts that the current supply is not sufficient, thanks. Typically, after a few days of what feels like endless nursing, the baby will go back to his previous pattern, but will be getting more milk at each feeding, as the increased milk supply is meeting his needs.

You can see why it's a problem when mothers react to these frequency days – as sometimes happens – by assuming they are no longer making enough milk for their baby and giving him a supplement instead. Now he'll be full, true, but instead of getting signals to make MORE milk, the breasts will fill up more and respond by making LESS milk. The baby gets more frustrated when he goes back to the breast because he was trying to increase milk supply, not decrease it. He tries to nurse even more often. The mother is more convinced than ever that something is wrong with her milk supply (why else would her baby be nursing all the time??), and increases the supplement. Her milk production drops even more. And soon her concern becomes reality, and she doesn't have enough milk to satisfy her baby. She would have, though, if she'd let her baby demonstrate his skill at increasing milk production.

Another possible cause is that the baby is coming down with an infection of some kind (or fighting one off) and trying to get as many antibodies and anti-infective factors into his system as possible. Many mothers have noticed that when a virus or illness is going through the family, the baby will start nursing very frequently.

Your Baby Is Not Lazy, Stubborn, Incompetent, or Rejecting You

Sometimes mothers who are having some difficulties breastfeeding are told – by nurses, midwives, friends, family, and others who are helping or supporting them – that their babies are lazy, or stubborn, or not trying. Sometimes mothers feel that their babies are rejecting them, that they refuse to take the breast because they don't like it, or don't want to breastfeed, or, worst of all, that they don't like their mothers.

NONE OF THESE THINGS ARE TRUE!

If you offer your baby the breast and he doesn't latch on, it's not because he's stubborn or lazy or mad at you. Or because there's something wrong with him. He's a baby. He is hardwired to breastfeed. Breastfeeding is so important to the survival of the human species that it couldn't possibly be relegated to something only "compliant and hard-working" babies do.

A baby who "won't" breastfeed can't breastfeed. It's not that he doesn't want to, he does. (Or he would if he was able to think that way. He'd want all the good things that breastfeeding offers – the closeness and comfort, the optimal development, the antibodies and immune support. But he doesn't know about those things. All he knows is that every cell in his body tells him to find the breast and get milk.)

So why can't he? Well, there are many possible reasons (Dewey, Nommsen-Rivers, Heinig, & Cohen, 2003):

- Medications given in labor may be affecting his abilities to find the breast, latch on, and coordinate sucking and swallowing. Breastfeeding, while simple in some ways, requires some complex abilities on the baby's part. It's as though you were given a dose of morphine, then asked to draw a complicated picture. You just can't do it.

- He's had some negative experiences and is trying to protect himself. Perhaps he had deep suctioning of his mouth and airways at birth and found that traumatizing – so he's avoiding opening his mouth at all. Or perhaps the first few times he was held in a breastfeeding position, someone pushed his (possibly sore from the birth) head into the breast, and he's afraid that will happen again.

- He's learned something different. Maybe his first feeding or two was given via a bottle. He's a smart kid. He quickly figured out that food comes from those firm plastic things, and that's what he's looking for when he's hungry. Now you offer him a soft, warm breast with a smaller, softer nipple. He thinks it's nice, but has no idea that this could also be a food source.

- There are some physical issues making breastfeeding hard for him. Some babies can't move their tongues effectively (tongue-tied); others have some pain or stiffness due to the birth. They need some help and patience to resolve these problems, so they can breastfeed successfully.

Your baby, right from the start, knows and loves you. Talk to him, even in a room with a dozen other voices, and he'll turn towards the sound of your voice. Express a little of your milk onto a breast pad, and he'll turn his head towards it rather than a breast pad with some other woman's milk on it. Yes, he does want to breastfeed. The job of people who are helping you with breastfeeding is to make it possible – not to criticize him or label him. He really is doing the best he can, and so are you.

What You Can Do Now

1. If you haven't yet done so, create a list of people who can help if you do run into breastfeeding challenges. Realize that sometimes you have to try more than one helper before you find the person who "clicks" with you and knows how to resolve your problems, so it's good to have a list.

2. Search on YouTube for videos of babies self-attaching ("breast crawl" is one description that is sometimes used). Be impressed by the amazing abilities of newborns!

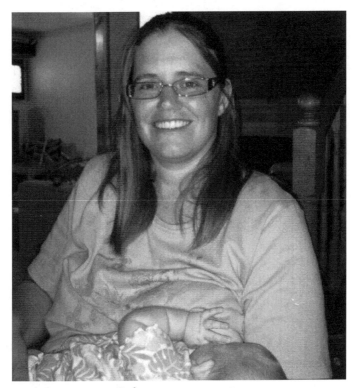

Chapter 6.
First Feedings

The moment you've been waiting for is finally here: Your baby is born. You get your first look at that beautiful (but possibly scrunched-up and covered with vernix) face and hear that little cry for the very first time. You're in love.

Ideally, the first feeding at the breast should happen as soon as possible after the birth and certainly within the first hour. Your baby is primed to breastfeed at this point and (unless you've had medications during labor) will be alert and ready. Until now, your baby was protected from germs by your body; but now that he's out in the big world, he needs the protection your milk can give him. The colostrum you are producing will give your rather vulnerable newborn a hefty dose of protective antibodies and immune factors, coating his digestive system so that germs can't get in, and adding a laxative effect to help clear the meconium from his intestines.

As well, breastfeeding is comforting and soothing to your baby who has just been through a dramatic change. As he nurses, he'll hear your familiar heartbeat and voice, be comforted by the touch of your skin, be soothed by suckling, and reassured that even though this new world he's entered is different, it is a very nice place to be.

First Feeding

So – here you are, with your baby. How do you start?

Ideally, neither you nor your baby should be washed before this first feeding, although usually the baby is dried off with a towel to keep him from getting too cool. Babies use their sense of smell to help them find the breast and washing can inhibit that. They also seem to follow the scent of the amniotic fluid on their hands as they move forward, so washing the baby should be avoided, too.

First, get yourself into a comfortable, semi-reclining position. If you are in a delivery room, you may be able to have a wedge behind you (or may already have one there), or you may be able to have the head and shoulders portion of the table cranked up a bit. If you are in a hospital bed, you can have the head of the bed made more upright – but not too much; you want to be reclined, not sitting up. (Sitting up at this stage may be pretty uncomfortable, even if you haven't had an episiotomy or tear, because your bottom is likely to be sore or tender.)

If you've given birth at home, you may want to get into bed and use pillows to get yourself into a comfortable position.

Sometimes a pillow or two under your knees, as well as the pillows around your head and shoulders, will be helpful, especially if you've had an episiotomy or a tear.

Now lie the baby down, skin-to-skin, on your body, with his head near but slightly below your breasts. If the room is cool, you may want a sheet or light blanket to cover you and the baby. Your body will keep him warm. Research shows that a mother's body will heat up as needed if the baby's body temperature is low and will cool down if the baby's temperature becomes too warm, much more effectively and efficiently than one of those "baby-warmer" units in hospital nurseries (Karlsson, Heinemann, Sjors, Nykvist, & Agren, 2012; Lunze & Hamer, 2012).

At first, he may just lie there, enjoying being close to you. You can talk to him, stroke him, even let the doctors or midwives examine him. He may cry a little, he may just be quietly alert, or he may doze off for a little while. In his own time, he'll start to move towards one breast or the other. Newborn babies have a natural reflex that allows them to push with their feet to help them move up your body. Sometimes it helps to put your hand under the baby's feet, so he can push against your hand.

As he gets close to the breast, he may bob his head up and down, searching for the nipple. His movements may look random at first, but if you watch, you'll see that he's getting closer and closer to his target.

You can help him as much or as little as you want or feel he needs. If your breasts are large, you may want to support the one he is moving towards. You may want a hand on his back and body to make sure he doesn't fall to the side. But be patient and let him go at his own pace.

At first, when he finds the nipple, he may just nuzzle or lick it. That's okay. When he's ready, he'll open his mouth wide and latch on. Usually the baby is on top of the breast and comes more or less straight down on the nipple. This helps to give a really deep latch, with the nipple well back in the baby's mouth. He may stay in this position – his face smooshed into your nipple and breast – or he may roll a bit sideways once he's latched on. Or he may not do the top-down latch at all, but come at the nipple from below, especially if you have larger breasts. There are lots of variations that can work – your baby will figure it out, maybe with a little help from you. The baby in the photo below is enjoying his first feeding.

Typically, the baby ends up diagonally across your body, his head higher than his feet. That's an easy position for you to give him a little support with your arms and hands. But if his position for this feeding is a bit different, don't worry. Over time you'll master nursing in many different positions!

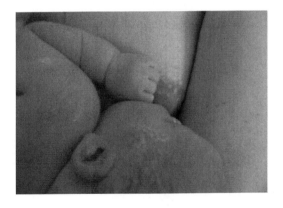

What If It Hurts?

Despite the many different approaches and positions babies use when they self-attach at the breast, they rarely cause any pain. But rarely doesn't mean never! If you feel pain when your baby latches on, try making some adjustments to see if you can get more comfortable without unlatching the baby and making him start over.

Your goal is to have the nipple as deeply in the baby's mouth as possible, so that he is getting a large mouthful of breast. It seems to be easiest to get this deep latch if the baby is covering more of the breast with his lower lip and jaw than with his upper lip and jaw. This is called an asymmetric latch. It works better because the only jaw we can actually move is the lower jaw, so this type of latch makes it easier for the baby to effectively compress the milk ducts with his tongue and lower jaw action.

So, if your baby has latched on and it feels painful, try to get a deeper and more asymmetric latch. How you do that will depend on your baby's position.

Let's say he's lying diagonally across your body, his head slightly to the side as he nurses. Try shifting him slightly down and pushing his shoulders a bit closer to you at the same time, without taking the nipple out of his mouth. Does it feel better? Remember you only need to make small changes – often getting the nipple a quarter of an inch deeper into the baby's mouth makes all the difference between pain and comfort.

Is he lying tummy-down on top of you, having come straight down on the nipple? This position is usually not painful, but it's possible that the baby hasn't gotten the nipple quite right in his mouth. Try moving him slightly down, towards your feet, to see if that helps. Or push up a bit on the bottom of your breast.

If all your efforts to wiggle into a better position seem to be not working, and the pain isn't subsiding, you can slide your finger into the corner of your baby's mouth and try again. It's best to only do this infrequently. Some mothers have been told to unlatch the baby and try again repeatedly, and this just makes the baby frustrated – every time he gets that nice breast in his mouth, somebody pulls him off and makes him start over. It's much better to adjust the positioning while the baby is nursing.

Sometimes the initial latch is painful, but the baby soon pulls the nipple into a better position and the pain goes away. In that case, don't unlatch the baby – but try to help him get a better latch right from the start next time.

Still hurting? Ask for a Lactation Consultant or another breastfeeding expert to give you a hand. It may be that your baby has some anatomical problem that is making breastfeeding painful and difficult, such as a tongue-tie or cleft palate. This should be checked out. No amount of adjusting position will resolve these issues. It may be that you have a yeast or bacterial infection on your nipples, or other physical problems.

What if the nurse or midwife notices that you are in pain, but tells you that it's normal for breastfeeding to hurt? You may have heard this from your friends as well. In fact, some women become quite offended if they are told that breastfeeding isn't supposed to hurt; to them, it feels like a criticism of their breastfeeding skills or at least of their experiences.

It's not meant as a criticism. Pain during breastfeeding is a sign of a problem. It doesn't mean the mother is doing something wrong or not trying hard enough. There are many different possible causes for this pain, and it may take some detective work to figure out what's going on. The mother deserves to get good help, so the pain can be relieved (if it's something that can be fixed – and usually, it can be). Pain is a common cause of early weaning, and often the weaning is unnecessary. If the mother had been able to get good help, the cause of the pain might have been identified and resolved.

So if your first feeding or feedings are painful, ask for help. Don't wait to see if it gets better or decide it's "not bad enough yet." You want to get the best possible latch, as early as possible, to help in establishing a good milk supply and making breastfeeding a positive experience for you.

Feeding Sitting Up

There are many benefits to using the laid-back breastfeeding position: It's comfortable for you, you don't have to support the baby's weight, and it creates the right environment for your baby to follow his natural instincts.

Sometimes, though, hospital staff feel strongly that mothers should breastfeed sitting up, or you may want to use this position for your own reasons. As your baby gets older and you are breastfeeding in different places and situations, you will probably want to be able to breastfeed sitting up (although you may still enjoy breastfeeding lying down or semi-reclining when you're at home). So here's how to take advantage of your baby's feeding instincts in that position.

Sit up, using pillows to support your lower back. You may want to have a pillow near your arm that you can slide into place if needed to help you support your baby once he's latched on. Hold your baby vertically, so his chest and tummy are against your chest. (It's ideal if you can be skin-to-skin, but babies can usually figure things out even if you have a shirt and bra on.) You should have one hand behind his shoulders and one behind his bottom.

Go ahead and talk to him and cuddle him. If he's hungry, he'll begin to bob his head (just as he does in the laid-back position), looking up at your face briefly, and then dropping down onto your chest again. He's orienting himself ("okay, face is up there, breasts must be just down here"), and in a few seconds or minutes will head towards one breast or the other. Some babies do this quite energetically, almost throwing themselves to the side, while others do it more gradually.

If your baby is not hungry, he will typically pull his knees up under his body, so his tummy is not against your tummy, and relax or go to sleep.

You should follow your baby's movement with your supporting hands and arms, helping him move to whichever breast he has chosen. (There is some evidence suggesting that the baby heads for the breast that is the 'most full' – perhaps the fuller breast smells more milky? We don't know.) You may need to provide some support for the breast, depending in part on how large your breasts are. To do that, shift your hands so that the hand and arm opposite to the breast your baby is aiming for are holding the baby – hand behind his shoulder, arm across his back. Use the other hand to support your breast in a position where the baby can easily get the nipple. (For example, if your nipple points straight down, you can put your hand under the breast and push the nipple up to make it more accessible for the baby.)

Continue to support the baby as he latches on. Usually, this will feel comfortable. If it doesn't, see if you can shift the baby's position a bit to make it feel better. It may help to move the baby slightly towards the center of your body, or to press his shoulders a little closer to your body, so his chin is buried more deeply in your breast. Remember, it doesn't have to be a big adjustment. The laid-back position is shown in the figure below.

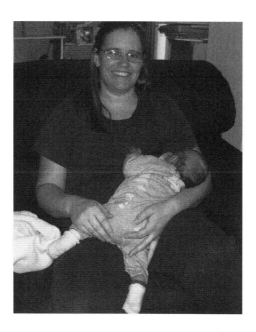

When Your Baby Needs More Help

Sometimes, for various reasons, babies need more help in latching on. You may find you need to hold your baby in a breastfeeding position (baby horizontally across your tummy, with one hand supporting your breast and the other hand supporting the baby's body). The hand that is supporting your baby's weight should be behind the baby's shoulders and neck, with most of the baby's weight on your forearm. Use the other hand (the one on the same side as the breast you are using) to stroke the baby's mouth or top lip with your nipple; this should encourage him to open his mouth wide. Once his mouth opens, you can bring him in closer by pressing his shoulders into your body as he latches on.

The Milk Came In!

Around day two or three or four, when your milk volume increases dramatically (and fluid from IV fluids may also come into play), you may find your baby is trying to latch on to very different breasts than just a few hours ago. Many babies take this in stride: They KNOW this is where the milk comes from, and they are determined that they are going to get latched on. Others react with some confusion and distress: What happened to that nice soft breast they were getting milk from yesterday? It's all different now! Help!

If you have edema (fluid in the breast tissue, not just extra milk), you can try a technique developed by Lactation Consultant Jean Cotterman, called Reverse Pressure Softening (RPS). Here's how you do it:

- First wash your hands.

- Then press back on the areola (the part of the breast with darker-colored skin around the nipple). By pushing back on this area, you will temporarily push the extra fluid back into the breast. You can do this by placing the tips of your fingers in a circle around the nipple, with the sides of your forefingers making a circle around the nipple, or you can use your thumb and forefinger. The goal is to create an indented circle of softer tissue that the baby can latch onto.

- Push in with your fingers and hold them there for about a minute. When you remove your fingers, the indented area should remain for a short time.

- Now quickly help your baby to latch on. If he's been latching well for the last few days, you should be able to do this fairly easily. If he doesn't get on and the indented area begins to fill with fluid again, you can do the Reverse Pressure Softening again.

- If you have a lot of milk, you can hand express some of it. This may make doing the RPS a bit easier. Avoid using a pump because the vacuum of the pump will pull more fluid into the breast tissue, creating more edema and swelling.

- You can use RPS every time you feed the baby, as long as you need to. The edema and engorgement should subside after a few days, especially if you are able to get the baby nursing well.

There's more information on this in the next chapter.

Using Breast Compression

Canadian pediatrician and breastfeeding expert Dr. Jack Newman was the first to teach mothers to use breast compression, but it was not his original idea. He saw mothers in Africa, where he was working, compressing their breasts as they fed their babies and asked them about it. They were surprised he didn't know about it and said that it helped the babies get more milk faster.

So what is breast compression and when should you use it?

It's a bit like hand expressing your milk into the baby's mouth, while he's nursing. To do it, you put one hand on your breast, with the fingers below the breast and your thumb on top, then squeeze the thumb and fingers together. You want to do this firmly, but not so hard that you bruise your breasts. Try not to slide your thumb down because you can irritate your skin, and this is more likely to cause bruising. The idea is just to squeeze or compress your breast between your thumb and fingers.

To know when to do this, you need to know how to tell when your baby is swallowing milk. It's harder in the first few days because the quantity of colostrum is fairly small, so you won't see the big gulps of milk. Typically, when a baby is nursing, he starts with a series of fast sucks: sucksucksucksucksuck. No real break in between them and no pausing when his mouth is open wide.

This helps to stimulate the breast to "let down" the milk that has been made and is waiting.

As the milk begins to flow, the baby's suck will change. Now you'll see: suuuuck, suuuuuuuck, suuuuck. In the middle of each suck, when the baby's mouth is open wide, you'll see a little pause. During that pause, the baby is getting a mouthful of milk. With colostrum, the pause may not be very long and you may not hear a swallow. But if you watch carefully, you can usually see the change.

After the baby does the slower sucking for a few minutes, the flow of milk typically slows down, and the baby goes back to the fast sucksucksuck pattern. Or, he may not suck as fast, but he's no longer pausing and swallowing.

That's when you use breast compression. By compressing your breast as the baby sucks (but when he's not getting a fast flow of milk, so isn't swallowing), you'll encourage another letdown and the baby will be rewarded with more milk. This can be quite helpful with a newborn who gets tired easily and may give up if he's not getting a lot of milk.

What You Can Do Now

1. Check out some of the videos on Dr. Jack Newman's website www.breastfeedinginc.ca/content.php?pagename=videos

These will clearly show you how to know when the baby is latched on well and swallowing milk. You might want to bookmark this site in case you have difficulties later.

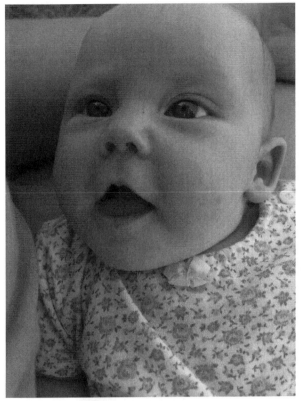

Chapter 7.
More Milk!

Usually around day three or four, sometimes earlier and sometimes later, the amount of milk you are making will increase dramatically. And when I say dramatically, I'm not kidding. For the first couple of days you are producing perhaps an ounce of colostrum from each feeding, but after this change, known in many places as "the milk coming in," you may find you are producing as much as five or six ounces at a time.

This is called "lactogenesis 2" because it is the second phase of milk production. The first (lactogenesis 1) started during your pregnancy, when you began making colostrum. Your pregnancy hormones prevented you from making more than a small volume of milk. Now those hormones are gone, and your body kicks into high gear.

The change happens quite rapidly and can be a bit startling for your baby. He latches on, expecting to get the slower-flowing colostrum that he got just a few hours before, and finds himself gulping down milk. Some are delighted; some are taken aback and may let go, getting sprayed in the face with your milk.

What may surprise you is how much bigger your breasts grow during this phase. That swelling is caused partly by an increase in milk and partly by increased blood flow and fluids in the breast to support the increased milk production. Your breasts may feel very full and firm, to the point of being painful. This is called **engorgement.**

If you had IV fluids during labor, some of that fluid will go into your breasts (as well as other parts of your body). This increases the painful swelling of your breasts and can make it very difficult for the baby to latch on. Sometimes the nipple almost disappears into the swollen breast. This swelling due to excess fluid is called **edema.** Edema and engorgement together can cause real problems for the breastfeeding mother and baby.

Preventing Problems When Milk Volume Increases

The two main things you can do to make this phase of breastfeeding easier are:

- Avoid interventions that require IV fluids during labor.

- From birth on, breastfeed your baby frequently, making sure he's latched on well.

As mentioned earlier, IV fluids in labor are absorbed into your body. Some goes into the baby's body, and some stays in yours. Over time, the fluid moves to your wrists and hands, feet and ankles, and breasts, causing the tissues to swell. (You will eventually pee it all out, but it can take several days.)

What interventions require IVs? Some hospitals encourage mothers to have an IV line hooked up as soon as they arrive in labor, just in case something goes wrong and the doctor wants administration of medication or another treatment where an IV line in place would be useful. It would save time in an emergency, the nurses will point out.

One alternative you can ask for, if routine IV is your hospital's policy, is a heparin lock. The nurse putting this in will insert a catheter tube, add a little heparin to stop the blood from clotting, and then close off the end of the tube. No fluids are going into your body, but the tube is ready in case it is needed to give you medicine or fluids later.

IV fluids are needed if labor is induced or sped up with the drug pitocin. If this kind of induction is suggested for you, ask about alternatives. Is induction really essential? Could you wait longer, while continuing to assess the baby? Are there other approaches to getting labor started that would be reasonable to try in your situation?

Women who have tested positive for Group B strep will normally be given antibiotics in IV fluids during labor in order to reduce the risk for the baby.

And IV fluids are also needed if you have an epidural. That's because an epidural can cause a significant drop in the mother's blood pressure; the added fluids keep your blood pressure from dropping too low. Of course, you'll also have IV fluids if you experience a Caesarean birth.

In any of these situations, minimizing the amount of time you have the IV in place can help to reduce the amount of fluids you are dealing with – and the problems they can cause for you. If you are getting antibiotics for Group B Strep, for example, ask if you can have the IV taken out as soon as you finish the last dose of the medication, rather than continuing on with it until the baby is born. If you are planning on having an epidural, consider waiting as long as possible (perhaps learning other ways to manage the pain of labor), so that you are getting the IV fluids for a shorter period of time.

On to part two of prevention – getting that baby to nurse well and often right from the start. For babies learning to breastfeed, it's all about practice. You want him to practice frequently, and you want to help him get it right each time. These frequent and effective feedings mean that as the milk volume starts to increase, the baby is already good at nursing. He'll be able to manage the extra milk that starts to flow, and he'll be able to work with the changing landscape of your breast as it fills up.

Problems with breastfeeding at this stage are often caused by a baby who really hasn't fed well in the first two or three days. He might have just taken the nipple in his mouth and sucked on it, not getting much milk, or he might not be opening his mouth wide enough to get part of the breast as well. While the baby is only getting a little milk, he's getting some, so he keeps on doing this. Then, the breasts become fuller and the nipple flattens out a bit, and suddenly baby can't latch on at all.

How you resolve this will depend in part on what is causing the breast fullness.

Engorgement

When the primary cause of breast fullness is engorgement – due to the milk volume increasing plus some natural increase in fluids in the breast to help with that kicked-up milk production – your main goal should be to get the milk moving to soften the breast and help the baby latch on.

You can use either hand expression or a pump to start this process. Sometimes a nurse or your midwife will show you how to hand express, but it's pretty simple if they don't. Put a cup or other container on a table (to catch any milk, otherwise this can be messy!). Put your thumb on top of your breast, and your other four fingers underneath. Your thumb should be near the edge of your areola, or roughly 1.5 inches back from the nipple. Gently but firmly squeeze your thumb and fingers together while at the same time pressing back towards your ribs. You should see drops of milk begin to appear at the end of your nipple. If you see nothing, try shifting your thumb and fingers slightly forward or backwards. The ducts in every breast are arranged a bit differently, and you will likely need to experiment a bit to find the best places to exert pressure and get milk. As you keep squeezing, you may see streams of milk spray out. That's good – you've found an excellent spot to apply pressure!

When you have expressed enough milk to soften your breast, especially around the nipple, try to latch the baby on. If he still can't latch, you may want to try a pump for a short time, as that may be more effective at bringing the nipple out.

Edema

If, on the other hand, much of the swelling in your breasts is caused by edema, you'll want to avoid using a pump. Why? The suction of the pump and the vacuum it creates can actually pull MORE fluid into your breast, making the swelling worse and not better. You may extract some milk, but the extra fluid can have the effect of making it harder for the baby to latch, and the pressure of the fluid against your milk ducts can reduce milk production.

How will you know if the fluid is mostly edema? Look for other signs in your body, such as swelling of your ankles and hands. You can also try gently poking your breast with one finger. Does that leave an indentation that goes away slowly? If so, you likely have edema.

One technique to help the baby latch is known as Reverse Pressure Softening, and was developed by Lactation Consultant Jean Cotterman. The idea is to push some of the fluid near the nipple deeper into the breast, so the baby has a soft area to latch on to.

There are several ways to do this. One is to use the four fingers of one hand and the four fingers of the other hand together to create a circle around the nipple with the fingertips touching the skin. Press down firmly and hold for 30 to 60 seconds. This should create an indented circle around the nipple. You can also apply pressure with the fingers of one hand, in a circle, or with your two forefingers placed horizontally around the nipple. As soon as you remove your fingers, help the baby to latch on.

Cabbage leaves (yes, ordinary cabbage) also help to relieve edema. To use these, remove the outer leaves of a head of cabbage and take off a few leaves from the next layer. Wash them well, dry them, and crush them slightly with your hands. Place them on your breasts (they should feel good because they are cool). Leave them there until they wilt, then replace with fresh ones. Don't overdo it, as you can decrease your milk supply with overuse. Cold compresses can also be used and research suggests both work equally well.

There are also foods that help you eliminate extra fluid (by peeing it out), so you might want to eat more of them: Cranberries, watermelon, celery, onion, and eggplant are some of the foods recommended.

Helping the Baby Latch

You've done what you can to reduce the swelling and get the milk flowing, but your breasts are still considerably bigger and firmer than they were just a day or so ago. How can you help your baby latch on? Try these tips:

- Even if you don't normally need to support your breast when your baby nurses, you may need to at this point, so that the heavier weight of the breast doesn't pull the nipple down and away from his mouth.

- You may also need to shape the breast to help the baby get a good mouthful. Think about how you might use your thumb and finger to flatten the front edge of a large burger so that you can get it into your mouth. The way you flatten the breast will depend on the position the baby is in as he latches on. If you are using a laid-back position and he is vertically on your body, you will start with your thumb held straight across the top of the breast (but back from the nipple) and your fingers supporting the breast from below. (If the baby is being held in your arms and lying on his side, your fingers and thumb should match the line of his mouth – going up the sides of the breast as they flatten it.) Squeeze your thumb and fingers together so that the breast is flattened, with the nipple sticking out in the middle. (Be sure your fingers and thumb are far enough away from the nipple that the baby can get plenty of breast into his mouth. Then latch the baby on. You can move your thumb and fingers back to continue supporting your breast as he nurses.

- Try a different position if your usual one isn't working. The football hold position, for example, puts your baby more underneath your breast, and gives you a bit more control of how he latches on (which can be helpful just now, although self-attachment is usually preferred). It also keeps the baby away from your other breast, which can help if you are really painfully engorged and wincing every time the baby kicks or accidentally hits your tender breasts.

- If you haven't tried it yet, the laid-back breastfeeding position may be a great option. Lying on your back can help drain any edema away from your nipples, especially if you add the Reverse Pressure Softening technique. Your baby will have gravity to help him get a deeper latch as well. See Chapter 5 for a full description.

When your baby does latch, you will probably hear gulping and obvious swallowing – all very good signs! If you don't, or if you're not sure if he's nursing well, keep an eye on his diapers. You should see his poops change from black, greenish, or brown to yellow within a day or two of your milk volume increasing.

Dealing With Discomfort

Yes, you want the baby to get on and get milk! But you also want your breasts to stop hurting! Some women, especially those experiencing both engorgement and edema, are in considerable pain during this stage. If the baby also has trouble latching well, you can add nipple pain to the breast pain, and you will soon be feeling pretty miserable and dreading each feeding.

What will help? Well, you can take over-the-counter pain medications, ideally those with anti-inflammatory properties. This will reduce some of the swelling, as well as the pain.

You can use both hot and cold compresses to make you feel more comfortable. Cold compresses can help to reduce the swelling and pain between feedings, but it helps to switch to hot compresses shortly before you think the baby will nurse again, because they encourage the milk to flow. Then switch back to the cold compresses after the feeding.

If your nipples are sore, you can apply an ice pack to them just before latching the baby on. That will temporarily numb them and reduce any swelling. For some women, cold makes their nipples turn white and throb painfully. If that's you, skip the ice packs!

When you do get the baby nursing, try to gently compress your breasts between your thumb and fingers. If that is painful, try massaging gently (you may want to use a little lotion first) from the top and sides of your breasts towards the nipple as the baby nurses. This may help get the milk flowing.

If you can, take baths rather than showers when you're dealing with engorgement. The water raining down on your breasts can feel like little knives stabbing into you! A warm bath may actually give you some relief – you may find you are leaking milk into the water.

If your breasts are large and heavy, a supportive bra may help you feel more comfortable. You may need one that is a cup size (or even two) larger than the bras you wore during your pregnancy. Look for a soft cotton type without underwires. You may be tempted to wear this at night while you are sleeping, but it's better not to because it's easy to get the bra twisted while you are asleep or pressing on a duct, and end up with a plugged duct or mastitis. A better option at night may be a fairly snug-fitting camisole or tank top, worn under your nightgown or pajamas, to give you some support without the risk of too much pressure in one area or another.

Leaking is often a major problem at this stage. You just have too much milk! Nursing pads in your bra or tank top can help soak up the leaks. Avoid getting the kind that have a waterproof plastic shield on the outside, as they will hold moisture against the nipple that can lead to irritation or even infection. And remember to change them frequently!

Waiting for the Milk

Not everyone sees their milk volume increase by day two or three. There are medical reasons why it sometimes takes longer, and other cases where there is no obvious cause for the delay.

What might delay the normal timing of the increase in milk volume?

- The mother is older than average.

- The mother is overweight.

- The mother has diabetes or high blood pressure.

- The mother is taking certain medications (such as SSRI anti-depressants).

- The mother had pain-relieving medications in labor.

- The labor was induced or augmented with pitocin.

- The birth was stressful or difficult.

- The birth was by C-section.

- The mother and baby were separated, or the baby did not nurse well or frequently.

- The mother has retained placental fragments.

This delay in milk coming in is a concern because often by day four the baby has lost a significant amount of weight and is clearly hungry and fussy. Frequently, the mother is advised to start supplementing the baby (and seeing her baby so unhappy seems like a very good reason to supplement), but this tends to lead to the baby spending less time at the breast and further delaying the milk coming in. It can also hamper the development of a good milk supply. Research shows a link between milk not increasing by 72 hours and early weaning – but, of course, the early weaning may actually be related to the supplementation, not any long-term breastfeeding problems caused by the delay in milk coming in.

About 98% of women will have their milk "come in" by seven days after the birth. (I have worked with a couple of mothers who waited ten days before the milk volume increased.) In the big scheme of things, that's not a long time – but when you have a hungry, cranky baby, it's endless.

If you notice that you have one or more risk factors (you are overweight and have high blood pressure, for example, or you are planning to use medications in labor, or have a scheduled C-section), you might want to prepare for this possibility by hand expressing and collecting some of the colostrum you produce during your pregnancy. You will only get a small amount at any one time, but you can cool that small amount in the fridge, then add it to the frozen milk you've already collected. You can start collecting colostrum as soon as you notice that you are leaking some or can hand express even a few drops.

Then, if your baby is getting hungrier, but you haven't yet seen the increase in milk volume, you'll be able to use the colostrum. Because the thicker colostrum isn't always easy to feed through a tube, you can add some sterile water to it, and then use a feeding tube at the breast to supplement the baby. By supplementing at the breast, you'll promote the milk coming in while keeping the baby fed – and with your own milk.

If you don't have colostrum to supplement with, and your milk is taking a long time to increase in volume, you may need to supplement with formula. Again, it works best if you can do this at the breast. If you can't, try to give the baby a small amount of supplement first, then put the baby on the breast to finish the feeding. It may help to pump or hand express after each feeding to encourage milk production.

Too Much Milk?

Most mothers worry about not having enough milk for their babies. But it's also possible to produce so much milk that the baby is spluttering and choking and struggling to cope with the fast flow. Often these babies are also fussy and have explosive, green poops.

This situation may just be temporary during the engorgement phase, but it can be a long-term problem for some women. If you find you are overflowing with milk by day three or four, try hand expressing or pumping briefly before you put the baby on the breast to get past the first overwhelming let down. Your baby may be able to manage the slower flowing milk after that.

If the problem continues after the first couple of weeks, though, you may want to talk to a La Leche League Leader or other breastfeeding expert. There are a couple of different approaches that can be tried, and you'll want to have someone help you figure out what will work best for you and your baby, without reducing your milk supply by too much.

What You Can Do Now

1. Buy a bra or two to wear during the engorgement stage. This bra should be a cup size or two larger than you are wearing while pregnant, and should be a soft, stretchy cotton type that gives good support, but doesn't have underwires. Ideally, you can pull the cup down to breastfeed. You might also want to get a snug camisole or tank top that you can wear at night.

2. Review the list of possible causes for a delay in the increase in milk volume. If one or more of these applies to you (or seems likely to you – for example, your doctor suggested that you may need a C-section), you may want to plan to collect and freeze some of the colostrum you produce towards the end of your pregnancy.

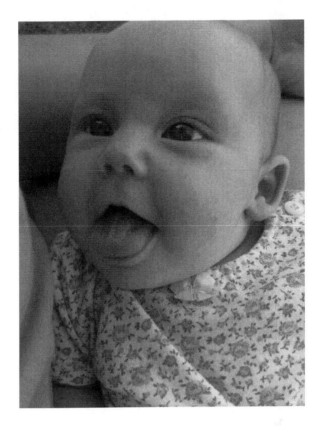

Chapter 8.
Supplementing

Most new mothers worry about having enough milk for their babies. Because they can't actually see how much milk is flowing into the baby, they wonder how much the baby is getting. What if he's starving?

Of course, what many don't realize is that not being able to see how much milk the baby is getting is actually one of the BENEFITS of breastfeeding. It means that the baby – and only the baby – is in control of how much milk he takes in. When you are using a bottle and can see that there is, say, a half an ounce left in the bottle, there is a strong temptation to coax the baby into drinking that last half-ounce. And because the milk will drip out of the nipple, even if the baby doesn't suck, he'll usually go along and drink it. That may not seem like a lot at the time, but those half-ounces add up (and, of course, sometimes it's more than half an ounce). And research suggests this can be a contributing factor to childhood obesity problems. At least one study has shown that toddlers who were given bottles when younger (whether the bottles contained formula or human milk) tend to finish any drink they are given, even if it is in a cup (Li, Fein, & Grummer-Strawn, 2010). Those who were breastfed without bottles tend to stop when they are done, whether there is more left in the cup or bottle, or not. The "eat everything on your plate" habit starts early.

All the same – it's a natural worry. So how can you tell if your baby is getting enough?

In the past, mothers were often advised to simply count the wet and poopy diapers. If it was coming out one end, it must have gone in the other end, right? Of course, that's true to a certain extent, but research has found that this really isn't reliable enough to count on. For example, a baby may have many wet diapers in the first few days because he has a lot of extra fluids on board from the IV fluids his mother had in labor. A baby who is gaining weight well and using most of the milk he gets may have only a few poopy diapers. Some babies will have a small bowel movement every time they nurse, others will have one or two large stools instead – so the count will be very different, but the overall volume is the same.

So, what do you look for? It's the whole picture that tells the story, not just one thing:

- Is your baby clearly swallowing and drinking milk for several minutes at each feeding? Do you see the change from the short, fast sucks to the long, slow sucks, with the pauses when the baby's mouth is open wide that indicate she is getting a mouthful of milk? This can be harder to see when your milk volume is still low, but you should definitely see it once the milk volume increases.

- In that first week, are the baby's poops changing in color from the black meconium to green, to golden brown, to yellow? They should be yellow and like thick pea soup in texture by day four. If not, ask for help with breastfeeding.

- What is the pattern of your baby's weight loss and gain? At first, all newborns will lose weight. Those who have absorbed extra fluid because their mothers had IV fluids in labor will lose more than those who have not. No worries, that's normal. By day four, though, the baby's weight should be starting to increase again, and you would expect the baby to be back to birthweight by about ten days. Of course, if the baby had a lot of IV fluids in his system, his birthweight will be inflated, and it may take longer to get back to that weight. What you are looking for is the pattern – is the baby gaining weight steadily at this point?

- And, finally, what are you seeing in the diapers? Is the urine clear (no dark yellow or orange urine)? That's a good indicator the baby is not dehydrated. Would the baby's poops (whether there are six or just two) add up to a handful over 24 hours? You don't have to actually hold them in your hand, just estimate. While not definitive, these are very good signs.

Being aware of all of these factors will help you know with some confidence that your baby is doing well.

What About Fussiness, Crying, Frequent Feeding?

Many mothers worry that their babies aren't getting enough milk, not because of problems with weight gain, but because of the baby's behavior. The baby nurses, doesn't go to sleep, and then wants to nurse again 20 minutes later. Or the baby does fall asleep, but wakes up showing obvious signs of hunger half an hour after that.

Or the baby often seems fussy and cries a lot, wanting to be held most of the time. Is he hungry?

The truth is that babies can be fussy for many different reasons. Some are just more sensitive than others – they cry when they are too cold, too warm, when the light is too bright, or just because they are missing you. Some seem to have digestive problems (possibly reacting to some food you are eating, but often just because their systems are not quite used to eating yet). Some are only happy if they are being held or are close to you. All these babies may be getting plenty of milk, but still be fussy.

Babies who nurse frequently in the early weeks may simply be doing what nature intended – establishing a good milk supply. Or you may be looking at a "cluster feeding," where the baby nurses several times over a period of a couple of hours, and then takes a longer break (perhaps sleeping for a couple of hours). This is a very common pattern for nursing babies.

In most cases, fussy babies are getting plenty of milk – or working to build up the milk supply.

But What If He Isn't Getting Milk?

The previous section described *most* babies. However, *some* babies are really not getting enough milk. How do you know?

- Lack of weight gain (or weight loss) is ultimately the most reliable indicator. However, you have to be sure to take into account the IV fluids that may be in the baby's system, and that the weights may be done on different scales. When you are weighing a baby, you are looking at very small amounts – if one scale is off by an ounce or two, it makes a big difference. I have known a number of situations where problems with the scale, or differences in calibration between scales, led to mothers being told their babies were not gaining well. So keep other indicators in mind as well.

- The baby's poops are still dark in color (blackish or greenish) after day four. His urine may be dark yellow as well, and wet and poopy diapers may be infrequent.

- Your baby nurses frequently, but you never see or rarely see those long, slow sucks with pauses that indicate he's getting mouthfuls of milk. Your nipples may also be sore.

- You haven't yet seen any increase in milk volume that is expected by day three or so.

Now what?

The first step is to see if you can improve the breastfeeding. In many cases where a baby is not getting enough milk, the mother is making plenty of milk, but the baby isn't getting it because he's not latched on well to the breast or is not feeding effectively. (Of course, over time this will lead to a decrease in milk production.)

- Have your baby's mouth checked by a breastfeeding expert, who will look for a tongue-tie, but will also check for any other anatomical problems. Babies with tongue-ties have the movement of their tongue restricted by the frenulum (the tissue that joins the tongue to the bottom of the baby's mouth), so they aren't able to efficiently extract milk. They will also make your nipples very sore! Releasing the tongue-tie is usually a quick and simple procedure, and the sooner it is done, the sooner breastfeeding will be going well.

- Ask for help with improving your baby's latch. If you've changed to sitting up or another position, try going back to the laid-back position described in Chapter 5. Ideally, have a breastfeeding expert watch what your baby is doing to see if the latch can be made deeper and more effective.

- Try using breast compression as the baby nurses. When the baby is sucking, but not swallowing, squeeze your breast between your fingers and thumb. This will encourage the milk to let down and flow, and you may see the baby begin swallowing. When the swallowing stops, let go, move your fingers and thumb a bit, and try again. When you no longer get any swallowing, even with compression, switch to the other breast.

If you feel that these changes are helping, but your milk supply hasn't quite caught up to baby's needs, try the "24 Hour Cure." This just means getting into bed with baby for 24 hours (or a whole weekend if you can manage it) to do nothing but nurse and snuggle. Keep baby in just a diaper, go topless yourself if you can, and nurse as often as the baby will nurse. Have someone bring you food and drinks if possible (if not, try to keep snacks and drinks handy in your bedroom). This relaxed time will often boost milk production and improve the baby's feeding techniques.

You've done all this and your baby still seems to be not getting enough? You might want to try galactagogues. These are herbs and medicines that increase milk production. There are many out there, some with research to support them, some just part of folk wisdom. The herbal supplement fenugreek does have some research (Turkyılmaz et al., 2010) to demonstrate effectiveness and is often used in combination with blessed thistle. There is also a prescription medication (Domperidone), available in some countries, but not the U.S., which is often very helpful. Eating oatmeal has also been shown to boost milk supply. If you are interested in trying any of these, talk to a Lactation Consultant or La Leche League Leader about the different options – some work better in different situations.

It's Still Not Enough...

Despite all their best efforts, some women will not be able to make all the milk their babies need. This can be very disappointing and frustrating, but the good news is that it doesn't have to mean the end of breastfeeding. You can continue to feed your baby at the breast while adding a supplement to meet the rest of his nutritional needs. Sometimes women only need to supplement for a period of time until their own milk production catches up. Many who supplement longer will be able to stop supplementing once the baby is eating solid foods, and just keep on breastfeeding.

The first choice in supplementing is to give the supplement at the breast. It saves time, keeps the baby interested in breastfeeding, and maximizes the mother's own milk supply.

Here's one way to do it:

- You'll need a small (four ounce) baby feeding bottle with a rubber nipple, a feeding tube (you can get these at medical supply stores), and some supplement, which could be milk you have pumped, donated milk from a milk bank or another mother, or formula.

- Use scissors or a small knife to widen the hole in the nipple, so you can put the feeding tube through the hole without compressing it. You want it to be held firmly in place but not squished.

- Pour the supplement into the bottle, put the tube in the nipple, so it extends to the bottom of the bottle when the nipple is screwed on, and screw on the nipple.

- Set the bottle on a table beside you (or stick it in your pocket) and latch the baby on. When he is sucking, you can gently slide the tube into the corner of his mouth, alongside your nipple. The end should be near the end of your nipple (you'll have to estimate how far to insert it, or measure against your other nipple and put your thumb at that point on the tube). His sucking will bring the supplement through the tube.

- Sometimes it works better to put the tube in place before you latch the baby on. You can use a bandaid to hold the tube in place on your breast if that makes it easier. Make sure the bandaid is high enough up on the breast that the baby won't be sucking on it.

Sometimes, especially if the baby is not doing well and gets very sleepy at the breast, mothers will insert the supplement tube at the beginning of the feeding. If the baby is doing well, though, you can start the feeding without the tube and watch him at the breast. If he is sucking and swallowing well, don't insert the tube right away. When he stops swallowing and is just doing the fast sucksucksuck, add the tube, so he gets the supplement. If your milk supply increases over time, you'll find you are inserting the tube later and later in the feeding.

You can also buy commercial kits for supplementing at the breast. Some allow you to put the supplement in a plastic bag that is attached to a strap you wear around your neck – this allows you to be more mobile and feed the baby more easily when you are out. Check out the different options and see what works best for you and your baby.

How much supplement should you give? With this system, the baby won't take more than he needs, so you can put a substantial amount in the bottle if you want – say, four ounces – but the baby may quit nursing after he's had an ounce or two. Then you can put in a bit less next time. As your milk supply increases, you'll find the baby is taking less supplement and you can adjust accordingly.

Other Ways to Supplement

Supplementing at the breast is the most effective way in terms of protecting breastfeeding and avoiding some of the problems linked to supplementation – research has shown that supplementation of breastfeeding during the first few days is a major factor in early weaning (Perrine, Scanlon, Li, Odom, & Grummer-Strawn, 2012; Dabritz, Hinton, & Babb, 2010; Gray-Donald, Kramer, Munday, & Leduc, 1985). But it's not always possible. Sometimes, for example, you may have a baby who isn't latching on at all. Or you may have been separated from your baby because of illness or other problems. So you'll need to find other ways to give him the milk he needs.

In the first few days, when the baby only requires small amounts of milk, the easiest method may be to use a spoon. You can hand express into a small, sterile container or directly onto the spoon. At this stage, if the quantity of milk you can get is still too small, you can add a little sterile water. If formula supplementation is necessary, it can also be given by spoon. It's easy to do: Support your baby in a sitting position in the crook of your arm, bring the spoon with the milk up to his lips and press gently on his bottom lip, then tip the milk in when he opens his mouth.

Another option is to use a syringe without a needle. You can insert the tip of the syringe into the baby's mouth, then slowly push down the plunger to give him the milk.

As your baby's need for milk grows, you can try cup feeding. Yes, babies can drink from cups - you have to help a lot, though! Support the baby in a sitting position in the crook of your arm, then hold the cup (it should be a small shot glass-size cup) full of supplement to his bottom lip. Tip in a little of the milk, so he gets a taste of it. At first, you may need to repeatedly tip in small amounts of milk, but he should soon get the idea and bring his tongue forward to lap up the milk instead.

If the baby is not latching, a technique called "finger feeding" can sometimes be used to help get the baby to the breast while giving some supplement. You would use a feeding tube and bottle just as for supplementing at the breast, but you tape (or hold, or use a bandaid) the tube to your finger instead. People usually use their pointer or middle finger for this. With the tube in place, you put your finger in your baby's mouth, and as he starts sucking, he'll get the supplement. After he's done that for a minute or two, you can try him at the breast. Because he's had a little bit of supplement (and so isn't frantically hungry) and has had some practice sucking, he may latch on.

Supplementing with Bottles

Some mothers, especially those who need to supplement long-term or those who are going to be away from their babies frequently (for work or school, for example), will decide to supplement with bottles. Because bottles are so common in our society, people often feel more comfortable using them in public situations than a tube-feeding setup at the breast, and baby sitters (or other family members who may be taking care of the baby) will usually want to use bottles.

One of the big risks with bottles, though, is that they often lead to weaning. Babies need to suck differently on the bottle than they do at the breast, and while some seem to go back and forth easily, others will have a hard time. It often seems easier for the baby to get milk out of the bottle than out of the breast (hey, it will drip out of the bottle if you hold it upside down – no effort required!), so the baby comes to prefer the bottle. This is especially true if the mother's milk supply is a bit low.

There are two strategies that can help with this and allow mothers to continue breastfeeding, even if they are supplementing with a bottle.

The first is *paced bottle-feeding*. This approach, described by Lactation Consultant Dee Kassing, is actually beneficial for the baby in several ways: It reduces the stress some babies experience with bottle feeding, and it helps the baby control how much milk he gets. It also may protect breastfeeding by making the baby work a bit harder by not getting large quantities of milk quickly from the bottle.

Here's how you do it:

- Support the baby in a sitting position. Hold the bottle in a horizontal position and offer it to the baby by touching the nipple to his bottom lip. If he's hungry, he'll take the nipple.

- By keeping the bottle horizontal, the baby has to actively suck to get the milk. Don't worry if the nipple has air in it – the baby will just burp it up.

- When the baby's sucking slows down or if the baby shows signs of wanting to take a break (starting to twist away from the nipple or pushing against the bottle with his hands), you can either tip the baby and bottle forward, so there is no milk in the nipple, or you can take the bottle out of the baby's mouth. Maybe burp him or just wait for a few moments before you offer the bottle again. Some babies will want several breaks during a feeding, others just one or two.

- Offer the bottle again, or move the baby back into the vertical position. If the baby is not interested – even if there is milk left in the bottle – stop the feeding.

As you get to know your baby, you'll get better at picking up the signs that the baby wants a break or is finished.

Part two is *give the supplement first*. I know that may be different from what you've heard, but let me explain. The usual approach for mothers who were supplementing breastfeeding in the past has been to breastfeed the baby first, then give the supplement; the idea was that you'd encourage the baby to take as much as possible from the breast before giving the other milk.

But in reality, what tended to happen was that over time the baby would spend less and less time breastfeeding, and be more and more interested in the bottle. Here's what we think was going on: The baby nursed at the breast, got some milk, but was still hungry. In his mind, the breast was not satisfying. Then, along came the bottle. Now his hunger was satisfied, and he got that contented, full feeling. Naturally, he starts to see the breast as something he has to get out of the way, so he can enjoy filling up on milk from the bottle, and some babies soon reject the breast completely.

If you give the supplement first, you reverse all that. Now the baby drinks from the bottle, gets a bit of milk, but is still hungry. Darn bottle! Not satisfying! Then he goes on the breast and gets filled up, and feels content and happy at the breast. He may stay on the breast longer because he's just enjoying being there, and he's less likely to reject it.

Of course, we can't really read babies' minds, but many mothers have had good success with the supplement first, breast second approach.

The trick is to give a little bit less supplement than you think is needed – you don't want the baby to be full. If it's not quite enough, no worries, he'll just be hungry a little sooner. It may take a little trial and error, and the amount of supplement may change over time, but those adjustments are not too hard to make.

Not Enough Milk? Not a Big Problem!

One of the most common reasons for weaning is not producing enough milk to meet the baby's needs. Yes, exclusive breastfeeding is preferred and is ideal in terms of baby's health and development, but you can still give your baby many of the good things about breastfeeding, even if you need to supplement. It can work and is well worth the extra effort.

What You Can Do Now

Talk to your doctor or midwife about local hospital policies on supplementation. Supplementing breastfeeding during the first few days is a major risk factor for early weaning and breastfeeding problems. It's good to be aware if the hospital has a high rate of supplementation and to discuss ways to minimize the risks to your baby.

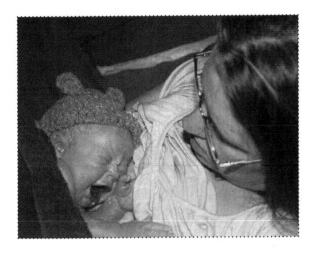

Chapter 9.
Life With A Breastfeeding Baby

It's hard to imagine before you have a baby what life will be like with a newborn to care for. Many of us get our ideas about new motherhood from TV shows and movies: The mother shows off the baby, maybe feeds it with a bottle, then announces, "time for a nap," and briefly leaves the set. No crying, no fussing, and she's back for the next scene a moment later. Looks pretty easy, doesn't it? Of course, what's really happened is that she just handed the baby to the mother.

But now, *you're* the mother! And as a breastfeeding mother, feeding the baby is pretty much your job, and it's a job with its own challenges and rewards.

Night and Day

One of the hardest parts about becoming a mother for many women is that it is 24/7. Every job you've ever had up until now probably had scheduled breaks, time for lunch, and a time to go home. Even if you had to work overtime, you got to go home at the end of the day and rest. If you had an especially crazy, busy week, you could sleep in or nap on the weekend to catch up.

Babies would not make good bosses. They are rarely predictable, they don't care that you are trying to eat lunch, and when you collapse into bed exhausted after a busy day of looking after them, they call you again. And again. If your baby was your boss, you'd be calling the HR department.

No question, it's not easy being responsible for a tiny new person around the clock. But there is good news, too. Breastfeeding helps you cope with the 24/7-ness of motherhood because:

- Breastfeeding helps you feel more loving and nurturing towards your baby when he cries (research shows that your brain actually responds differently than the brains of mothers who are not breastfeeding). You don't mind going the extra mile when it's for someone you love as much as you love this little guy.

- Breastfeeding is less work: All you have to do is lift up your shirt or unhitch your bra and let the baby nurse. You can be relaxing on the couch, lying in bed, or cuddling with your partner at the same time. No preparing formula, heating up bottles, washing bottles and nipples, or running to the store for more. You have all you need.

- Breastfeeding makes you feel more relaxed and positive, researchers say. This helps you get through the stressful times (and there will be some).

For those frequent daytime feedings, it can help to set up little "nursing stations" in different parts of your home. You don't want to have to always retreat to the bedroom when your baby's ready to nurse again. So pick a few spots (the bedroom, of course, but also a couch where you can watch TV or be on the computer, a comfy chair by a window, or anywhere else that appeals to you) and equip them with diapers and baby wipes, receiving blankets or burp cloths, and maybe a bottle of water or a snack for you. A pillow or two in each spot to help you support the baby if needed can be useful, too.

As your baby gets older and both of you master the techniques of breastfeeding, you might find a baby sling helpful because you can put the baby in the sling, latch him on, and deal with any household tasks you need to do.

Mentally, it can help to NOT look at the time or try to count how often the baby has fed (unless, of course, you are having some breastfeeding problems and the Lactation Consultant or La Leche League Leader you are working with has asked you to keep track). I say that because I've seen many women who tell me they are feeding the baby "on demand" or "on cue," but who still have in their minds the idea that a baby should only eat every three hours or every four hours, or some other schedule. In fact, it's very normal and typical for a baby to eat irregularly – perhaps three feedings in two hours, followed by a longer break, and then three or four more feedings in close succession. By eating in this way, the baby meets his own variable needs and also maintains good milk production.

When you are checking the clock, though, it's easy to think, "but he can't be hungry again! He just ate an hour (or two hours, or thirty minutes) ago!" The truth is he might be hungry, or he might be needing more antibodies, or he might be trying to boost or increase your milk production, or any of a dozen other things. Or, he might just need some comfort and closeness, something else that breastfeeding is very good at providing!

At night, it may help to minimize what you have to do. Who wants to get up and walk down the hall to retrieve a crying, hungry baby? If you keep your baby close to you at night, you'll get more rest; having your baby in the same room at night also reduces the risk of SIDS.

What about bedsharing? Many public health groups have campaigns against bedsharing, suggesting that it increases the risk of the baby suffocating or dying unexpectedly. Other researchers say that bedsharing can be safe, providing certain factors are present (Ball, 2003). The factors that make bedsharing safer are:

- Breastfeeding

- Mother is sober (i.e., not taking any medications or drugs that would impair her awareness, and not so exhausted that she's unaware of the baby's presence)

- Non-smoking (and also did not smoke while pregnant)

- Sleeping on a safe surface (i.e., not a waterbed or very soft mattress, no heavy duvets, etc.)

The bedsharing baby should sleep next to his mother, and research shows that she will naturally and instinctively arrange herself in a safe position as they both sleep. The baby will usually roll onto his back as he finishes breastfeeding, which is the safest way for a baby to sleep.

Unfortunately, many mothers who hear the anti-bedsharing campaigns assume that beds are dangerous – so they sleep with their babies on couches or recliners, which are known to be MUCH more dangerous than beds. Or they try to sit up on a chair at night to breastfeed, only to find they are so tired they can't stay awake (and the relaxing hormones of breastfeeding certainly don't help you stay awake!). Babies have been injured, and even killed, when their mothers fell asleep and let them roll off their laps.

Hormones (and Periods and Sex)

During the time you are breastfeeding, the hormones circulating in your body are a bit different from those of the non-breastfeeding mother. One thing those hormones can do is suppress your menstrual cycle. When you are exclusively breastfeeding in response to your baby's cues, you are not likely to have your period (and if you do, you will probably not be ovulating). It is possible, though, to ovulate before that first period returns.

Women do vary quite a bit in this, and some will have their periods return within a few months of giving birth, while others will go two years or more if they continue breastfeeding. On average, among women who breastfeed into the toddler years, their periods return at about 14 months. Breastfeeding does help reduce your chances of becoming anemic (not having enough iron in your blood) because of those menstrual periods that you DON'T have (not to mention the savings in tampons, pads, etc.).

Wait – does that mean you can't get pregnant if you are breastfeeding? No. In fact, there are many, many women who have conceived while nursing another child. On the other hand, breastfeeding can prevent pregnancy under certain circumstances:

- Your baby is younger than six months old.

- You are breastfeeding exclusively (no bottles, no pacifiers, etc.).

- Your periods have not returned.

When all three of these conditions are present, your chances of getting pregnant are very low. As soon as you change one of them, though, the risk of pregnancy starts to go up. At this point, you might want to use temperature/mucous charts to determine whether or not you are ovulating and to see how your cycles are changing, or you might want to use another form of birth control.

The same hormones that suppress ovulation can also suppress your sex drive. This can be discouraging if you've been looking forward to having things "get back to normal" after the sometimes weird hormones of pregnancy (and after your doctor or midwife has given you the go-ahead to resume sex). And it's hard to know what to blame on hormones and what to blame on the state of exhaustion that almost every new mother exists in. Having a nap seems WAY more appealing than having an orgasm.

Not only that, on those occasions when you do feel rested enough and interested in a little loving, thanks to your hormones you may find you have much less vaginal lubrication than usual. Painful sex is not going to make you look forward to the next time, so be patient with yourself. If you and your partner can spend more time on the "warm-up" phase, maximizing the amount of lubrication you produce, sex will be more enjoyable. You might also want to try some of the artificial lubricants you can buy. (Still not really comfortable? Well, this might be a good time for some alternative types of sexual activity...)

Your interest in sex will come back. I promise. It's important that your partner knows you're not rejecting him or her, that this is simply the result of hormones that keep you focused more on mothering than sex. Look for ways to show your love and affection, and experiment to see what kinds of activities will satisfy both of you.

Leaking

In the beginning, your breasts may seem rather...incontinent. They may start to leak milk if you see your baby, hear your baby cry, smell your baby, think about your baby, have a shower, hear another baby cry, accidentally rub your nipple, etc., etc. Leaking can be unexpected and annoying. Leaking can also happen during sex play or orgasm, so keep a couple of towels handy during those activities, too.

What can you do? If you feel the milk starting to let down, try crossing your arms over your breasts and pressing down firmly. This may stop the leaking. Other than that, your main strategy is preventing everyone else from noticing. There are several different kinds of breast pads on the market that will absorb the milk; you just tuck them inside your bra (or inside a snug camisole or tank top if you don't wear a bra). Many are disposable; others can be washed and re-used.

Some have a plastic coating or lining on the outside to make sure the milk doesn't leak through. This can be helpful if you are going out in public and are really concerned about possible leaks, but these plastic-lined pads really shouldn't be worn routinely. They hold the moisture in against the nipples and can cause soreness from irritation or an overgrowth of candida (yeast). If you do use these pads, be sure to change them frequently, so most of the time they are dry.

Wearing patterned tops can help disguise any small leaks; you might also want to wear or bring with you a light jacket that you can put on if needed to hide the wet circles.

The good news about leaking is that it usually diminishes considerably after a few weeks, and then stops most of the time. Of course, if you miss a feeding or go longer than usual without feeding the baby, you may experience some leaking.

Some women do have to deal with leaking longer than others. If it is an ongoing problem for you, you might want to talk to a Lactation Consultant. It may be that you have an oversupply of milk and might benefit from some strategies to reduce it. Or you might find it helpful to breastfeed more frequently, so you are not as full between feedings.

It's All You: Comfort, Food, Sleep

When you are pregnant, you are everything to your baby: his source of food, oxygen, warmth, life. When you are breastfeeding, especially in those early weeks, your baby still relies on you for most of the necessities of life, even though he's no longer inside your body. You are his source of food, his best comforter, his safe place to sleep, his familiar home.

While there's something lovely about that, it can also feel overwhelming to a new mother. Why is all this responsibility on YOUR shoulders? It's the kind of thing the feminist movement fought against with the slogan "Biology is not destiny."

And that slogan is perfectly true today, with formula and bottles and nannies and daycare, mothers don't have to take on the full responsibility for their babies' needs. But while biology is not necessarily destiny, it is still significant. Breastfeeding is all about biology! Breastfeeding is easiest and most likely to work when mothers and babies are together most of the time, and when the baby is brought to the breast whenever he's hungry, sad, or in need of comfort.

We've found ways to stretch that biology a bit (with pumps and galactogogues, etc.), but it can only stretch so far.

Your baby learned to recognize your voice, heartbeat, and even your smell before he was born. Your breasts provide not just food, but all those familiar things, as well as the warmth of your body and the comfort of your touch. Remember Harlow's experiments with monkeys? They clung to the soft, cuddly "mothers," even though it was the unpleasant and uncomfortable wire "mother" that provided food. Breastfed babies get both – the food and the cuddling all at once. No wonder your breastfeeding baby develops a strong attachment to you.

Entire books could be – and have been – written on the topic of attachment. It's a hugely important part of a child's development. Sometimes breastfeeding mothers worry that their babies are "too attached" to them because they protest when the mother leaves the room or fuss if someone else tries to hold them. A baby can't be "too attached." In fact, the standard description for a good, secure, desirable attachment in a one-year-old baby is that the baby protests or cries when the mother (or person the baby is attached to) leaves, and is happy and comforted when the mother returns. When your baby wants only you, that's not bad – it's a sign he's developing exactly as he should!

Sounds good, but that doesn't always make it easier. Maybe you'd just like to have a bath alone, or get back to the gym, or have a date night with your partner, and you're feeling frustrated that your baby isn't cooperating and always wants you, you, you. What can help? Here are a few ideas:

- Try to identify what you really need. Are you longing for adult conversation with your partner? Could it work to order in a nice meal and rent a movie, then relax together once the baby falls asleep? Do you just want to get some exercise? Could you take a brisk walk with baby in a carrier or wrap, or use a jogging stroller?

- Can you trick the baby a little? You want a bath all by yourself, but your baby doesn't sleep well without you there. Grab a T-shirt or nightie that you've worn, but not washed, and wrap the baby in it. Your familiar scent may help keep her calm and asleep.

- Look for things you can do WITH your baby: Go to a La Leche League meeting to get to know other mothers; head for "diaper days" events at the movie theater to watch the films you want to see without worrying that others will be annoyed by your baby's noises; seek out family-friendly and breastfeeding-friendly restaurants.

When you are in the middle of this stage, it seems like it will go on forever. Really, it doesn't. By six or seven or eight months, your baby will start eating solid foods and crawling around – the first steps towards independence. She might be quite happy to eat banana slices with Daddy while you head out for a bike ride or work on your novel.

Picture a timeline for your entire life – let's say it's 20 inches long, representing 80 years. Each year is then marked out as a quarter of an inch. Those six months when your baby's need for you will be most intense are only one-eighth of an inch. That's all: one-eighth of an inch, a little sliver of time, in 20 inches. It really is just a tiny part of your entire life, but so important for your baby's future health, development, and well being. There will be time for the other things.

When You're Sick

You wake up in the morning feeling woozy. A hand on your forehead confirms it: You have a fever. You feel queasy, maybe you even throw up. Or you start sneezing and coughing. Whatever the symptoms, you know you're sick. But you're also breastfeeding. Now what?

Every mother dreads these days, but they happen. You'll catch a cold or a tummy bug, or something worse, and you feel horrible. Being sick was bad enough before baby arrived, but now you have new responsibilities, and you need new strategies:

- Keep breastfeeding! Are you concerned about passing on the virus or illness to your baby? Don't be. You are usually most contagious before you have any symptoms, so your baby has already been exposed to whatever illness you have. Stopping breastfeeding now won't protect him. What it will do is deprive him of the antibodies and immune factors that your body is making and adding to your milk – factors that can protect him from getting the illness or reduce the severity if he does get sick. He needs your milk now more than ever. Continued breastfeeding also helps prevent you from developing plugged ducts and mastitis.

- Drink more. If you have a fever, vomiting, or diarrhea, you are at risk of becoming dehydrated anyway – add breastfeeding to that, and your risk is even higher. Take small but frequent sips of water or water with electrolytes added. If you do become dehydrated, contact your doctor.

- Get help if possible. If you can find a friend or relative who can tend to the baby and you, but still bring the baby to you when it's time to nurse, that will make a big difference.

- No help available? If your baby isn't mobile yet, snuggling into bed together may be the best strategy. You can rest and nurse frequently, and the baby will be safe and close by.

- Check any medications your doctor recommends or that you are considering taking to see if they are compatible with breastfeeding. A La Leche League Leader can look them up for you in one of her resources. You can also check Lactmed or Motherisk online, or the book *Medications and Mothers' Milk* by Dr. Thomas Hale.

If you are so sick that you are not able to take care of your baby at all, or need to be in the hospital, you might want to see if you can arrange for a breast pump (even if the nurse or another person has to actually pump your breasts for you). Abruptly stopping breastfeeding may mean you end up with mastitis, and since your body is already trying to fight off one illness, that can make your situation even worse. Pumping through your illness also means it's more likely you'll be able to go back to breastfeeding, even if the baby had to have bottles while you were ill.

When Baby Is Sick

What if your baby is the one who is sick? Yes, breastfeeding does reduce the risk of babies becoming ill, but it doesn't eliminate all risk, and your baby may come down with anything from a mild cold to a more serious disease.

Your first sign that he's sick may be that he starts nursing more often than usual. He's attempting to stock up on antibodies and immune factors to help get rid of whatever germs have invaded his body. Even if he is vomiting or has diarrhea, it's okay – even desirable – to continue breastfeeding. Your milk is rapidly absorbed, so he'll get some nutrition, even if he throws up a few minutes later. And, perhaps most important, nursing will comfort and soothe him when he's feeling miserable.

Out and About With Baby and Nursing in Public

One study found that for more than half of the women who opted to use formula rather than breastfeed, concerns about breastfeeding in public were a major factor in their decision (Shortt, McGorrian, & Kelleher, 2012). Maybe it's something you've worried about, too. Will you get harassed or criticized for breastfeeding in a public place? Will people stare or make comments?

North American society has some odd attitudes about breasts. It's common to see women in clothing that reveals most of their breasts, and models in low-cut tops are popular for advertising everything from beer to cars. That's largely accepted. But the breastfeeding mother may get rude comments or be asked to leave.

In most places, you have the legal right to breastfeed wherever you and your baby are allowed to be.

Still feeling a bit awkward about the idea? Here are a few tips:

- Practice latching your baby on in front of a mirror, so you'll see how little skin is actually exposed and can figure out the easiest approach.

- You may want to have some "nursing in public" clothes. One option:

Get a tank top that fits fairly snugly and cut two openings where your breasts are. You can wear this under a shirt or T-shirt to minimize the amount of skin that's seen when you feed the baby. Another option: Wear a loose-fitting open jacket or cardigan over top of your shirt or T-shirt, so you can pull it forward to cover you and your baby at the breast.

- You can also check out some of the clothes designed for breastfeeding in public with hidden openings.

- What about the cover-ups sold for use while breastfeeding? I'm not a fan. These tend to call attention to the fact that you are breastfeeding, and many babies hate them (especially when it's warm) and will push the extra fabric away. But if you like them, experiment at home first to see if your baby will tolerate the covering.

- Choose your location. In a restaurant, for example, you may feel less exposed if you sit with your back to most of the restaurant; a booth can give you more privacy if you want it.

- Smile! If you look confident about what you are doing, people will be less likely to give you a hard time or make comments. Remind yourself that you have every right to be there and that you are doing the best for your baby.

Postpartum Depression

About 10% of women experience postpartum depression, but a much higher percentage experience "the baby blues" – feelings of sadness and hopelessness that aren't severe enough to be called depression, but that can make life pretty miserable all the same.

Wondering if this is affecting you? It's normal to have some ups and downs when you have a new baby – the changes are pretty overwhelming, after all – but here are some signs that you might be experiencing postpartum depression:

- Loss of appetite

- Insomnia

- Intense irritability and anger

- Overwhelming fatigue

- Loss of interest in sex

- Lack of joy in life

- Feelings of shame, guilt, or inadequacy

- Severe mood swings

- Difficulty bonding with your baby

- Withdrawal from family and friends

- Thoughts of harming yourself or your baby

    (From the Mayo Clinic website: www.mayoclinic.com/health/ postpartum-depression/DS00546/DSECTION=symptoms)

These symptoms need to last for more than two weeks to "count" as true depression, but if you are feeling this way for even a few days, you may want to talk to your doctor or midwife and discuss treatment options.

New research has suggested that postpartum depression (and other types of depression as well) may be linked to inflammation, and may be helped by supplements of Vitamin D and Omega-3 Fatty Acids.

Many women who are experiencing the baby blues or postpartum depression are advised to stop breastfeeding. The thinking behind this recommendation is that breastfeeding is adding stress to the mother's life. If she weans the baby, someone else can feed it and take care of it, and the mother can get more rest or can do other activities that may help improve her depressed feelings.

However, research has found that when breastfeeding is going well, breastfeeding mothers are less depressed than mothers who are not nursing. In fact, just putting your baby to your breast can make you feel better. Breastfeeding also protects the baby. When mothers are depressed, their babies tend to have abnormal brain development (because the mothers do not interact with them as they normally would). The babies of depressed breastfeeding mothers, though, have normal brain development.

If your doctor suggests taking antidepressants, you can ask that he or she prescribe one that is compatible with breastfeeding (many are).

Note that the research mentioned above talked about "when breastfeeding is going well." When you are having problems, you may end up with sore nipples, plugged ducts, and other problems that can cause inflammation – and inflammation is linked with depression. So this is yet another reason to seek out good help as soon as possible if you are running into any difficulties with breastfeeding.

Postpartum depression is also less likely if you have good support as you make the adjustments to your new life as a mother. Don't have a lot of family and friends to help out? You may be able to arrange for a postpartum doula to help look after you (and your household) during the early weeks after you have a baby.

And be kind to yourself. You've just done an amazing thing – made a new human. You deserve to take it easy and relax.

Colic

Having a colicky baby can both break your heart and make you furious. You feel so bad for your baby who is crying, crying, crying... and then you reach the point where you just feel angry and want to scream at her: STOP CRYING!

We don't know the underlying causes of colic, but it seems that in all societies around the world there are babies who cry more than others. Dr. Ron Barr, one of the leading researchers on this topic, says that one difference between North American parents and parents in tribal societies he has studied is that the tribal parents respond to their babies' cries very quickly – within seconds. North American parents often wait a few minutes. With colicky babies, that waiting means the baby gets much more worked up and cries much longer. He also found that carrying the baby in a baby carrier (or wrap or sling) can cut the amount of crying in half. The trick is to carry the baby throughout the day, not just after the crying has started.

Some parents have found draping the baby over the forearm to be helpful. The pressure on baby's tummy seems to offer the baby relief. The baby is being held in the colic hold in photo below.

Babies who are fed formula are more likely to have colic than those who are breastfed. That makes sense: Formula (despite all the advertising of "comfort proteins") contains many components and chemicals that a baby's digestive system is not really designed to handle. Some breastfed babies who are colicky are actually reacting to something in their mothers' milk. Common offenders are caffeine, dairy products, soy products, eggs, citrus, and wheat (Lust, Brown, & Thomas, 1996). You don't have to eliminate all of those at once, but try eliminating one at a time to see if there is a difference. 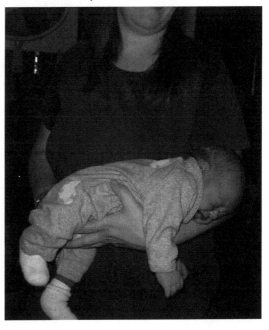 In one study, more than half of the colicky babies improved dramatically when their mothers stopped consuming dairy products (Jakobsson & Lindberg, 1983).

So what do you do with a colicky baby? Offer the breast first. Sucking is very soothing to babies, and if the problem is gas or an unsettled tummy, nursing can help to "move things along." Your baby will hear your voice and heartbeat, and have the comfort of being skin-to-skin with you. Even if he just nursed recently, he may be happy to suck and be soothed on an almost-empty breast.

But sometimes that won't work. When your baby is crying inconsolably, Dr. Barr recommends you try "contact, carry, walk, and talk." In other words, hold your baby (skin-to-skin can help even more) as a first step. If that doesn't work, try carrying him (in a carrier or in your arms), go for a walk or dance with him, and talk or sing to him as you move. These four components tend to be very soothing to babies.

The best thing about colic is that it usually ends, all on its own, at about three months. I know that can seem VERY far away when your baby is just three weeks old and crying all the time. But knowing that it will end, you can call in as many friends and family members as possible to give you a hand, cuddle the baby when you're too tired, take the baby for a walk so you can nap, or anything else that will get the two of you through these challenging weeks.

Your Partner and Your Breastfed Baby

Many women decide that they'd like to share the task of feeding the baby with their partners. They want to introduce a bottle early on (filled with either pumped milk or formula), so both parents can participate equally.

This works for some families; others find it quickly leads to early weaning from the breast (for reasons discussed elsewhere). If formula is used in the bottle, the baby is exposed to some of the risks of formula feeding as well; if pumped breastmilk is used, that means a lot of extra work for the mother who is breastfeeding some of the time and pumping to provide milk for the bottles.

It can be hard for the other parent who sees the deep, primal connection between the mother and breastfeeding baby. Bottlefeeding can't duplicate that, though. If preserving breastfeeding is important to both of you, it may work better for the non-breastfeeding parent to develop a relationship with the baby that isn't dependent on giving food. In fact, that's a good role to have – showing the baby that love isn't necessarily related to eating.

Babies need to be fed, sure, but they need lots of other things that don't need to come from "the one with the milk-filled breasts." They need to be carried, cuddled, changed, bathed, entertained, played with, talked to, shown the world, sung to, tickled, rocked to sleep, soothed and comforted, burped, and many more things.

You don't have to be the mother to do any of the items on that list. Dad and baby are skin-to-skin in the photo below. Both seem quite content.

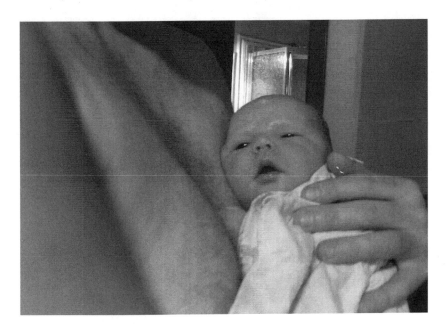

But the other parent also has a hugely important role to play in supporting breastfeeding. Researchers say that when partners are encouraging and positive about breastfeeding, the mother is likely to keep going; if partners are negative, the mother will wean. Support goes beyond just the words you say:

- Bring drinks, snacks, even the TV remote control, when she's nursing the baby.

- Give her a shoulder and back massage – even a seven-pound baby starts to get pretty heavy when you're carrying him so many hours a day.

- Defend her against negative comments from others (especially if the others are members of your family!). Let them know that breastfeeding is what you have chosen, that you support her, and that you believe it is the best thing for your baby and your family.

The most important thing parents can do when they have a new baby (breastfeeding or not) is keep the lines of communication open. This is a stressful time; both of you will be feeling overwhelmed and dealing with many changes in your lives. It's easy to feel hurt by things that are said or done (or not done) during these times, but taking the time to talk about how you feel and what you need from each other will help prevent those hurt feelings from growing into something worse.

What You Can Do Now

1. Check out the laws in your state or province that govern breastfeeding in public. It can boost your confidence to know that you are legally entitled to breastfeed wherever you need to!

2. When you are out and about, notice which restaurants and stores make mothers feel welcome. Notice which places encourage mothers to breastfeed (perhaps with signs saying "breastfeeding is welcome here"), have breastfeeding lounges, and have baby-changing stations.

3. If you haven't yet, make a list of groups you may want to check out that can provide support once your baby is here. Make sure La Leche League is on that list!

4. Talk to your partner about how he or she sees your growing family. How does your partner imagine building a relationship with your baby? How can you support that? What kind of support for breastfeeding are you looking for from your partner?

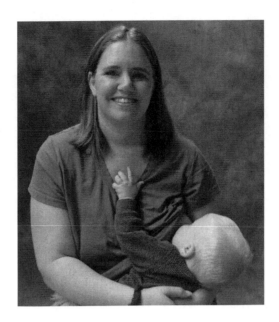

Chapter 10.
Your Breastfeeding Goals

You've got the information to get breastfeeding off to a good start. What now?

What are your goals for breastfeeding? Do you plan to follow the recommendations of the World Health Organization and most pediatric associations: Exclusive breastfeeding for the first six months, adding solid foods after that, with continued breastfeeding to two years and beyond? Or are you thinking you'll breastfeed for six weeks or three months, then wean and return to work (if you live in the U.S.)? Or are your plans to breastfeed for a year (while you're on maternity leave), and then breastfeed evenings and weekends as you go back to work.

Getting a solid foundation in breastfeeding will make it easier to achieve your goals, whatever they are. You may also find they change as time goes on. It's hard to even imagine nursing a toddler when you have a newborn at your breast, but it often seems perfectly natural once your child reaches that age.

Breastfeeding Through Separations

Obviously, breastfeeding is easiest when you and your baby are together. But many women today are working or attending school, and many have found ways to keep breastfeeding going despite these separations.

Sometimes women think they'll have to wean when they return to work, but that's rarely the case. Even if you aren't able to pump at work, you can usually continue breastfeeding during the times you are at home. Breasts can adjust to many different schedules, and even to changing schedules.

Entire books have been written on breastfeeding and working (including books on breastfeeding and special situations, such as women in the military), but here are a few tips:

- It's worth the effort to ensure you get off to a good start. Remember that effective, frequent nursing (or milk removal) in the early weeks helps to establish milk production for the entire duration of breastfeeding. Having a solid milk supply early on will give you more flexibility later.

- Take as much time as you can to be with your baby. Depending on your job and where you live, you may not have many options, but if you can add on (for example) some unpaid leave, or some vacation time, etc., this may help you make sure breastfeeding is going well before you have to return to work.

- Don't be in a rush to introduce a bottle. It's not true that the baby MUST be given a bottle before a certain age or he'll never take one. If he does resist taking the bottle when he goes to day care, he can get milk in other ways – with a cup or spoon, for example. You may find, at least at first, that your baby won't drink much while in day care, but will nurse frequently in the evening and overnight. This "reverse cycle feeding" is very common.

- If you are going to pump your milk, try to find a pump that has flanges in different sizes, because the fit is very important. You need to be able to create a good seal with the flange against your breast, but not have it be so tight that it hurts or bruises your breast.

- Human milk that is frozen loses some of its immune properties. It is still more appropriate for a baby than formula (which never had those immune properties to begin with), but it's not quite as good as fresh milk. So, if you are pumping for your baby, it's better to keep the milk refrigerated. Human milk can be safely kept in the fridge for five days, so just feed it to the baby within that time.

- Of course, many mothers like to maintain a stash of frozen milk for those days when they are too busy and haven't had time to pump.

If you have a changeable schedule (for example, some nurses work twelve-hour shifts that may sometimes be during the day, and sometimes at night), you may find it challenging to match your baby's needs. Sometimes, if you don't have time or a good spot to pump, you may want to hand-express some milk to keep yourself comfortable and to maintain some milk production, even if it has gone down. You can experiment and find out what works for you and your baby – and sometimes that will mean giving formula as well.

Early Weaning

Maybe you've decided that you want to stop breastfeeding after a few weeks or a few months. It might be because of the demands of work, family factors, or just because you want to stop. How do you go about it?

Babies are designed to breastfeed for two years and beyond, as the World Health Organization states. But a day, a week, a few months of breastfeeding all give your baby very significant benefits. You can feel proud of yourself no matter when you wean.

The key to mother-led weaning (as opposed to weaning that the baby instigates) is to do it gently and lovingly. That's easier on both you and the baby than a "cold turkey" approach, and it helps you remember that breastfeeding means more to your baby than just getting food – it's also a source of connection to you and a way to be comforted and soothed.

If you are weaning a young baby, you will probably want to give the baby bottles of formula. The easiest way to start is to pick a time of day when the baby is least interested in nursing – perhaps mid-morning. Offer the bottle then, in a playful way. If the baby seems to dislike the taste of the formula, you may need to make those first bottles with your own milk.

Once the baby is used to having one bottle of formula a day, and your breasts are no longer feeling full at that time of day, choose another feeding to replace with a bottle, and so on. Typically, a baby's favorite feedings are those before bedtime and/or naptime, and the one first thing in the morning, so mothers usually leave those as the last feedings to drop. By that point, your milk production should have decreased, and your baby should be showing interest in the bottle.

Remember that you're not just replacing a source of milk – you need to think about ways to keep the connection between the two of you and provide the comfort that breastfeeding once did. What can you add to your daily routine or interactions with your baby that will make that work? Rocking the baby in a rocking chair helps sometimes, using the sling or baby carrier more can help too. Perhaps you could learn baby massage techniques to provide more soothing touch.

You should also know that if you change your mind at any point and want to continue nursing – perhaps with fewer feedings per day – you can. It's entirely up to you and your baby. Some mothers have weaned completely for several weeks, then changed their minds and gone back to breastfeeding. It's not always possible, but it's been done.

As Your Baby Grows

As your newborn becomes a baby and eventually a toddler, your nursing relationship will change. At first, a baby is totally focused on breastfeeding; the entire house could fall down around you, and your baby would still be suck,

suck, sucking away. As she gets older, there will be more interaction: She'll look up at you and smile as she nurses (the nipple still in her mouth), she'll reach up and give you a free dental examination while nursing, or she will reach across and touch your other breast. By four months or so, many babies are easily distracted by the sights and sounds around them, so breastfeeding can be a series of short periods of sucking, followed by letting go to look around and squeal at people, more sucking, turning away from the breast to see what that noise is (often without letting go of the nipple!), more sucking, etc. Some mothers in busy households have resorted to nursing in a darkened bathroom with the water running to block out other noises.

Once your baby is mobile, you'll find breastfeeding is often a quick "touching base" behavior. Your baby will be excited to explore the world, but will want to frequently come back to you for a quick session of "na-nas."

Speaking of na-nas: If you are planning to breastfeed past the first year, it can help early on to choose a word to refer to breastfeeding that won't embarrass you if your child yells it out during dinner with the grandparents or at the shopping mall. Many will pick words like "na-na" or "nur" if you use the word "nursing." Choosing words like "milkies" and "boobies" can make others (and you) feel uncomfortable.

The Breastfeeding Parent

Breastfeeding teaches you a lot about parenting. When you breastfeed, you are learning right from the start to recognize your baby's cues, so you know when he's hungry. You're respecting his own inner wisdom about how to breastfeed, when to feed, and when he's full. This understanding of your baby will stand you in good stead as he grows up and you need to meet his needs in other ways. Breastfeeding can help you see your baby's uniqueness and individuality.

Breastfeeding can help you as you get started in mothering because it encourages your brain to respond to your baby in a loving and nurturing way. Then you build on that as your relationship grows and changes.

One day, your baby will wean (or you will encourage weaning). It's really the first of many weanings and changes in your relationship that you'll have throughout your life together. Learning to get through these changes while maintaining your close and connected relationship is important; the lessons you've learned while breastfeeding can help.

Everything I Needed to Know I Learned by Breastfeeding

1. Mother nature really does know best.

2. If it hurts, something is wrong.

3. People, especially very tiny people, are more important than things.

4. You have more power to love than you ever thought you did. Your heart, like the Grinch's heart, will grow a couple of sizes every time you have a baby.

5. Nobody really needs eight hours of uninterrupted sleep.

6. If you can't help someone who is crying, at least you can be there for them.

7. Pay attention. It may keep you from being bitten.

8. Go with the flow.

9. Touch heals, comforts, and is as essential as food. Get as much as you can.

10. When you have grown a baby inside your body, given birth, and watched that baby grow at your breast, you know you can do anything.

References

Alexander, J.M., Grant, A.M., & Campbell, M.J. (1992). Randomised controlled trial of breast shells and Hoffman's exercises for inverted and non-protractile nipples. *BMJ, 18*, 304(6833), 1030-1032.

Arora, S., Vatsa, M., & Dadhwal, V. (2008). A comparison of cabbage leaves vs. hot and cold compresses in the treatment of breast engorgement. *Indian J Community Med., 33*(3), 160-162. doi: 10.4103/0970-0218.42053

Australian Breastfeeding Assocation. (2012). Breastfeeding with large breasts. Retrieved from: http://www.breastfeeding.asn.au/bfinfo/large.html

Ball, H.L. (2003). Breastfeeding, bed-sharing, and infant sleep. *Birth, 30*(3), 181-188.

Ball, H.L., Ward-Platt, M.P., Heslop, E., Leech, S.J., & Brown, K.A. (2006). Randomised trial of infant sleep location on the postnatal ward. *Arch Dis Child, 91*(12), 1005-1010.

Canadian Institute for Health Information. (2013). *Childbirth highlights*. Retrieved from: https://secure.cihi.ca/free_products/Childbirth_Highlights_2010-11_EN.pdf

Centers for Disease Control and Prevention. (2012). *Breastfeeding report card – United States, 2012*. Retrieved from: http://www.cdc.gov/breastfeeding/data/reportcard.htm

Childinfo. (2013). *Statistics by area/child nutrition*. Retrieved from: http://www.childinfo.org/breastfeeding_madagascar.html.

Dabritz, H.A., Hinton, B.G., & Babb, J. (2010). Maternal hospital experiences associated with breastfeeding at 6 months in a northern California county. *J Hum Lact, 26*(3), 274-285. doi: 10.1177/0890334410362222

Dewey, K.G., Nommsen-Rivers, L.A., Heinig, M.J., & Cohen, R.J. (2003). Risk factors for suboptimal infant breastfeeding behavior, delayed onset of lactation, and excess neonatal weight loss. *Pediatrics, 112*(3 Pt 1), 607-619.

Gray-Donald, K., Kramer, M.S., Munday, S., & Leduc, D.G. (1985). Effect of formula supplementation in the hospital on the duration of breast-feeding: A controlled clinical trial. *Pediatrics, 75*(3), 514-518.

Health Canada. (2012). *Breastfeeding initiation in Canada: Key statistics and graphics (2009-2010)*. Retrieved from: http://www.hc-sc.gc.ca/fn-an/surveill/nutrition/commun/prenatal/initiation-eng.php

Ingall, M. (2006, December). *The breastfeeding myth*. Retrieved from: www.babble.com.

Jakobsson, I., & Lindberg, T. (1983). Cow's milk proteins cause infantile colic in breast-fed infants: a double-blind crossover study. *Pediatrics, 71*(2), 268-271.

Jørgensen, M.H., Ott, P., Juul, A., Skakkebaek, N.E., & Michaelsen, K.F. (2003). Does breast feeding influence liver biochemistry? J *Pediatr Gastroenterol Nutr. 37*(5), 559-565.

Karlsson, V., Heinemann, A.B., Sjörs, G., Nykvist, K.H., & Agren, J. (2012). Early skin-to-skin care in extremely preterm infants: thermal balance and care environment. *J Pediatr. 161*(3), 422-426. doi: 10.1016/j.jpeds.2012.02.034

Karlström, A., Lindgren, H., & Hildingsson, I. (2013). Maternal and infant outcome after caesarean section without recorded medical indication: findings from a Swedish case-control study. *BJOG*, 120(4), 479-486. doi: 10.1111/1471-0528.12129

Kellymom.com. (2012). A comparison of breastfeeding rates by country. Retrieved from: http://kellymom.com/fun/trivia/bf-rates-2004/

Kim, P., Feldman, R., Mayes, L.C., Eicher, V., Thompson, N., Leckman, J.F., & Swain, J.E. (2011). Breastfeeding, brain activation to own infant cry, and maternal sensitivity. *J Child Psychol Psychiatry*, *52*(8), 907-915. doi: 10.1111/j.1469-7610.2011.02406.x

Kramer, M.S., Aboud, F., Mironova, E., Vanilovich, I., Platt, R.W., Matush, L.,…Promotion of Breastfeeding Intervention Trial (PROBIT) Study Group. (2008). Breastfeeding and child cognitive development: New evidence from a large randomized trial. *Arch Gen Psychiatry, 65*(5), 578-584.

Li, R., Fein, S.B., & Grummer-Strawn, L.M. (2010). Do infants fed from bottles lack self-regulation of milk intake compared with directly breastfed infants? *Pediatrics, 125*(6), e1386-93. doi: 10.1542/peds.2009-2549

Loftus, J.R., Hill, H., & Cohen, S.E. (1995). Placental transfer and neonatal effects of epidural sufentanil and fentanyl administered with bupivacaine during labor. *Anesthesiology. 83*(2), 300-308.

Lucas, A., Morley, R., Cole, T.J., Lister, G., & Leeson-Payne, C. (1992). Breast milk and subsequent intelligence quotient in children born preterm. *Lancet*, 339(8788), 261-264.

Lunze, K., & Hamer, D.H. (2012). Thermal protection of the newborn in resource-limited environments. *J Perinatol, 32*(5), 317-324. doi: 10.1038/jp.2012.11

Lust, K.D., Brown, J.E., & Thomas, W. (1996). Maternal intake of cruciferous vegetables and other foods and colic symptoms in exclusively breast-fed infants. *J Am Diet Assoc, 96*(1), 46-48.

Mangesi, L., & Dowswell, T. (2010). Treatments for breast engorgement during lactation. *Cochrane Database Syst Rev,* Sep 8;(9), CD006946. doi: 10.1002/14651858.CD006946.pub2

Marks, L.R., Clementi, E.A., & Hakansson, A.P. (2012). The human milk protein-lipid complex HAMLET sensitizes bacterial pathogens to traditional antimicrobial agents. *PLoS One, 7*(8), e43514. doi: 10.1371/journal.pone.0043514

Mok, E., Multon, C., Piguel, L., Barroso, E., Goua, V., Christin, P., … Hankard, R. (2008). Decreased full breastfeeding, altered practices, perceptions, and infant weight change of prepregnant obese women: A need for extra support. *Pediatrics, 121*, e1319-e1324.

Nikodem, V.C., Danziger, D., Gebka, N., Gulmezoglu, A.M., & Hofmeyr, G.J. (1993).

Do cabbage leaves prevent breast engorgement? A randomized, controlled study. *Birth, 20*(2), 61-64.

Noel-Weiss, J., Woodend, A.K., & Groll, D.L. (2011). Iatrogenic newborn weight loss. *Int Breastfeed J,* 6(1), 10. doi: 10.1186/1746-4358-6-10

Penn, A.H., Altshuler, A.E., Small, J.W., Taylor, S.F., Dobkins KR, & Schmid-Schonbein, G.W. (2012). Digested formula but not digested fresh human milk causes death of intestinal cells *in vitro*: Implications for necrotizing enterocolitis. *Pediatric Research, 72*(6), 560-567.

Perrine, C.G., Scanlon, K.S., Li, R., Odom, E., & Grummer-Strawn, L.M. (2012). Baby-friendly hospital practices and meeting exclusive breastfeeding intention. *Pediatrics, 130*(1), 54-60. doi: 10.1542/peds.2011-3633

Sheehan, D., Krueger, P., Watt, S., Sword, W., & Bridle, B. (2001). The Ontario Mother and Infant Survey: Breastfeeding outcomes. *J Hum Lact, 17*(3), 211-219.

Shortt, E., McGorrian, C., & Kelleher, C. (2012). A qualitative study of infant feeding decisions among low-income women in the Republic of Ireland. *Midwifery, Nov 8*. pii: S0266-6138(12)00043-5. doi: 10.1016/j.midw.2012.03.001.

Swain, J.E., Lorberbaum, J.P., Kose, S., & Strathearn, L. (2007). Brain basis of early parent-infant interactions: Psychology, physiology, and in vivo functional neuroimaging studies. *Journal of Child Psychology and Psychiatry,48*(3-4), 262–287.

Szabo, A.L. (2013). Review article: Intrapartum neuraxial analgesia and breastfeeding outcomes: Limitations of current knowledge. *Anesth Analg, 116*(2), 399-405. doi: 10.1213/ANE.0b013e318273f63c

Turkyılmaz, C., Onal, E., Hirfanoglu, I.M., Turan, O., Koç, E., Ergenekon, E., & Atalay, Y. (2011). The effect of galactagogue herbal tea on breast milk production and short-term catch-up of birth weight in the first week of life. *J Altern Complement Med,* 17(2), 139-42. doi: 10.1089/acm.2010.0090

Tveit, T.O., Halvorsen, A., & Rosland, JH. (2009). Analgesia for labour: A survey of Norwegian practice – with a focus on parenteral opioids. Acta Anaesthesiol Scand, *53*(6), 794-799. doi: 10.1111/j.1399-6576.2009.01988.x

VBAC.com. (2013). *CDC reports most women receive epidural or spinal anesthesia for labor pain.* Retrieved from: http://www.vbac.com/2011/04/cdc-reports-most-women-receive-epidural-or-spinal-anesthesia-for-labor-pain/

Watson, J., Hodnett, E., Armson, B.A., Davies, B., & Watt-Watson, J. (2012), A randomized controlled trial of the effect of intrapartum intravenous fluid management on breastfed newborn weight loss. *J Obstet Gynecol Neonatal Nurs, 41*(1), 24-32. doi: 10.1111/j.1552-6909.2011.01321.x

Index

About the Author

Teresa Pitman has been working with pregnant women and breastfeeding mothers for more than 30 years. She's a La Leche League Leader, a childbirth educator, and a doula who has shared her knowledge and experiences in books and magazine articles. Her most recent books include *The Womanly Art of Breastfeeding 8th edition* (with Diane Wiessinger and Diana West) and a newly-revised edition of *Dr. Jack Newman's Guide to Breastfeeding* (with Dr. Jack Newman). She is a frequent speaker at conferences. Teresa is the mother of four grown children and the grandmother of five, with grandchild number six expected this spring.

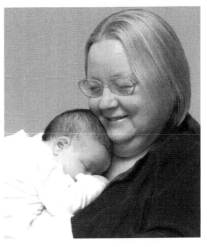

Ordering Information

Hale Publishing, L.P.
1712 N. Forest Street
Amarillo, Texas, USA 79106

8:00 am to 5:00 pm CST

Call » 806.376.9900
Toll free » 800.378.1317
Fax » 806.376.9901

Orders
www.ibreastfeeding.com